# Slow Viruses

# Slow Viruses

**David H. Adams**
Medical Research Council
Demyelinating Diseases Unit
Newcastle General Hospital
Newcastle upon Tyne, England

**Thomas M. Bell**
Department of Virology
Royal Victoria Infirmary
Newcastle upon Tyne,
England

**1976**
**Addison-Wesley Publishing Company**
Advanced Book Program
Reading, Massachusetts

London · Amsterdam · Don Mills, Ontario · Sydney · Tokyo

ISBN 0-201-00042-3
ISBN 0-201-00043-1 (pbk.)

Reproduced by Addison-Wesley Publishing Company, Inc., Advanced Book Program, Reading, Massachusetts, from camera-ready copy prepared by the authors.

Printed in the United States of America

ABCDEFGHIJ-HA-79876

PREFACE

One of the major and probably fairly exceptional problems
we have encountered in our attempt to write an essay on slow
viruses is the almost complete absence of any solid body of
accepted evidence which could be used as a basis.   In the
first place it has been necessary to try to make our own
definition of both the topic and the area involved.

We have for example begun from the conclusion that if the
term 'slow virus' is to be meaningful it must be restricted
to viruses which are 'slow growing' (or 'slow replicating'),
and consequently that the term 'slow virus diseases' should
properly apply to diseases resulting from infection with slow
growing viruses.   The reasons for this view will be given in
the early part of this volume.   We have also tried, because
it seemed essential, to begin from both the disease standpoint
and that of fundamental principles of viral replication and
to direct the two lines of thought towards common ground.
Although to a greater or lesser extent it is always difficult
to bridge such a gap it has become more and more obvious to
us during our enquiries that the gap in this case is very

large.    It seems quite clear in fact that any better understanding of slow viruses and the mechanisms associated with
them will depend on the ability of future investigators to
extend the boundaries.

The clinical symptoms of the slow virus diseases tend
to be ill defined and variable, particularly in the early
stages, and while much has been written about the associated
pathological changes they are not always clearly reconcilable
with the clinical symptoms.   Also, many of the biochemical
and virological considerations have of necessity been extrapolated from first principles by a combination of experience,
educated guess work and sheer speculation.   Bearing all this
in mind, we hope that it will be understood that it is a
daunting problem to attempt to integrate the biochemical,
virological, cell-virus relationship and disease aspects of
slow viruses.   Particularly in a volume of this size we
realize that at best we can do little more than scratch the
surface.   We make no apology therefore for the fact that
this volume has an unusually high content of personal
opinion, and we accept that some at least of our views will
be considered controversial.   All that we can say is that
we have made an honest and painstaking effort to deal with
the slow virus problem as we see it, in as many aspects as
possible, and in an overall way which does not seem to have
been attempted before.   We hope that the blunders, errors
and omissions which we have no doubt made will at least be
measured against the difficulties involved.

We also hope that what we have written will help others,
not only to learn something, but also to recognise the problems and pitfalls which beset the study of these fascinating
infective agents.   Particularly we hope that some may be

stimulated to take up the challenge - and to do better!

## ACKNOWLEDGEMENTS

We are most grateful to many colleagues for helpful discussions. Particularly we thank Professor P. S. Gardner and Dr. H. M. Wisniewski for reading and commenting on the manuscript.

We are also grateful to the Editors of Pathologie-Biologie and the Biochemical Society for permission to reproduce Figures 2 and 3 respectively.

CONTENTS

Chapter

Chapter

CHAPTER 1

INTRODUCTION

Over the last 20 years a multitude of review articles
has appeared covering virtually all aspects of the nature,
composition, structure and mechanism of replication of
viruses.  However, the experimental studies on which these
have been based have largely centred on a few fast acting
common viruses.  Recently, an increasing amount of work
has been directed towards a small group of infective agents
whose most obvious characteristic is that they are unusually
slow growing.  In comparison with the fast growing viruses
our knowledge of the nature and properties of these slow
infective agents is fragmentary and it is not even entirely
accepted at present that they are 'viruses' in the classical
sense.  However it is becoming more and more urgent  to try
to begin to find answers to the problems posed by them
because it is clear that they are the cause of an ever
widening number of rare, but unusually severe diseases.
Apart from their intrinsic interest in this respect, one of
the major questions which arises is 'why are they slow'?
So far as we can see, current literature provides few direct

1

clues because despite wide coverage of the work on almost
all aspects of virology virtually no attention seems to have
been given to parameters which may govern the rates of viral
replication and the lengths of the time interval between
infection and the appearance of viremia or disease.

We shall begin on the tacit assumption that the slow
(growing) infective agents probably are 'viruses' in the
classical sense, but with special properties.  Because of
present divergencies of opinion (48, 78, 80) we will attempt
to make an exclusive definition of what is meant by the
terms 'slow virus' and 'slow virus disease' in relation to
other virus groups and diseases.  Then we shall examine the
steps involved in the replication of classical virus
particles (virions) to determine their potential ability for
rate limitation, in an attempt to see how 'slowness' might
arise.  We shall next consider the properties of a typical
slow virus (that producing the disease of scrapie) in the
light of conclusions drawn from the classical viruses.
Finally, we shall consider the implications of 'slowness'
for the disease producing capability of the viruses involved
and conclude with a primarily clinical description of the
definite and putative individual slow virus diseases of man.

The time interval between infection and appearance of
viremia or disease - defined as the 'incubation period' -
may in general be divided into two relatively rapid phases.
During the first phase, the latent period, little or no
active virus is produced.  The second phase - which may
begin quite suddenly - is that in which viral replication
occurs, and this may be followed by a recognisable disease
state.  In most instances, and fortunately for the host,
the second phase is followed by an equally rapid decrease in
virus titer and recovery.  Although typically the whole

process occupies only a few days and rarely extends beyond
a four week period, it is nevertheless quite clear that a
minority of viral agents do not fit this pattern and, if
viral agents are taken as a whole, then both latent periods
and rates of replication in the infected tissues vary
enormously.

At one end of the scale lie such agents as the murine
virus, first discovered by Riley as a contaminant of transplanted tumors, which has the interesting property of
elevating plasma lactate dehydrogenase activity in infected
animals, but without causing any obvious disease.   After
intraperitoneal inoculation into mice this virus remains
latent for a period of about 6 hours, and then a rapid
viremia develops.   The plasma concentration increases 10
fold (1 $\log_{10}$) every hour for the next 10 to 11 hours, and
then decreases more slowly by about 5 logs over the next two
to three weeks.   At the other end of the scale, in mice
inoculated intracerebrally with the infective agent of
scrapie, the titre in the brain remains almost unmeasurable
for 2-4 months and then increases by 1 log/10-20 days for a
further 3-6 months.   These time periods are very approximate
for the development of scrapie and may be influenced in many
ways which will be dealt with later.   There is no decrease
in agent titre at any stage, except perhaps shortly before
the death of the animal, which occurs usually about 6-12
months after inoculation.   In sheep, the natural scrapie
host, the time course of the disease can be even longer, with
the period between infection and death extending to as much
as three years.

It may be pointed out here that 'slowness' per se is by
no means an unknown biological phenomenon, and diverse
examples can be given.   Some seeds take a long time to

germinate and the time required for germination may be
increased by subjecting them to adverse conditions such as
storage.    Carcinogens may not produce malignant growth for
very prolonged periods - twenty years or more in some cases
in man.    Diseases ascribed to genetic defects may not make
their appearance until late in life, and although it may be
said that the eventual disease has always been present but
without showing itself, the evidence for such a conclusion
is often poor or non-existent.

So far as viruses, taken in their entirety, are concerned a whole spectrum may be plotted of the incubation
periods between infection and onset of disease or peak of
virus titer (Fig. 1).    The great majority of the common
viruses of which examples are given in Fig. 1 do in fact have
short incubation periods, and consequently lie towards the
left hand part of the Figure.    Incidentally, it is
important to remember that the majority of the individual
lines in Fig. 1, designating the members falling within this
short incubation period, cover a larger or smaller group of
more or less closely related viruses - as many as 40 in
some instances.    As one proceeds towards the right the
number of examples sharply decreases, and it becomes more
uncertain how many variants there are in each.    Moving even
further to the right there is an amorphous collection of
'latent' viruses which remain apparently inactive in their
hosts for an indefinite period.    How many there are in this
group we do not know - partly because they are difficult to
detect - but they may be very numerous.    They must, of
course, be differentiated from viruses which, after
infection, disappear from, or are eliminated by, their hosts.
The essence of latency is the continuing presence in the
host of virus, or at least of viral components, which are

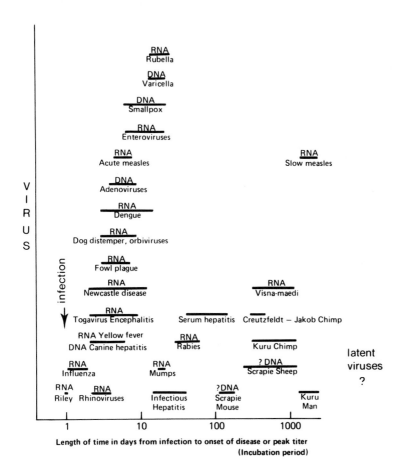

Fig. 1
The lengths of the incubation periods (the time between infection and disease or peak viremia) for different viruses. The approximate range of the incubation periods for each virus or group of viruses is given by ———— . The nature of the core material (RNA or DNA) is stated for those viruses in which the information is available.

potentially capable of replication - rather like a seed kept
in conditions which are unfavourable to germination.   How
many such agents are completely latent in the sense that
they do not replicate at all, and how many could, but have
no chance to do so because their latent period is longer
than the lifetime of their host, is an open question.
Some latent viruses may come to light only because their
replication is 'triggered' by other events which 'help'
latent viruses to emerge - such as the infection of their
hosts by other, active, viruses, or alteration of the hosts'
immune status.

       As with the length of the incubation period, it is also
clear that viruses can be arranged in a relatively continuous
spectrum concerning their effects on individual cells in
culture.   Some (lytic) agents rapidly fill the host cell
with new particles until it 'bursts' and releases its
contents, while others produce a range of more or less
subtle morphological changes, in some cases without causing
cell death.   Many latent, persistent and slow virus
infections cause either no or very slight cytopathological
effects, even after a prolonged period.

       In summary then, the spectrum of virus incubation periods
in their host animals runs a course from the very fast
acting agents to those whose replicative ability is virtually
zero under the circumstances applied to them.   Slow viruses
may be provisionally considered as those with exceptionally
long incubation periods, which possibly merge into the
'latent' group in the way mentioned above.   Also, for the
moment let us assume that 'slow viruses' are the cause of
'slow virus infections', although as will be seen
subsequently the tendency to equate these two terms has
caused a good deal of confusion.

# CHAPTER II

## DEFINITION OF SLOW VIRUSES

The idea that 'slow virus' diseases formed a distinct group was first put forward by the late Bjorn Sigurdsson in 1954 (17) and he defined them in terms of the following criteria:-

1. A very long initial period of latency lasting from several months to several years.
2. A rather regular protracted course after the appearance of clinical signs, usually ending in serious disease or death.
3. Limitation of the infection to a single host species, with anatomical lesions occurring in only a single organ or tissue system.

One difficulty which arises over Sigurdsson's original list is that the disease nomenclature which he used has changed over the intervening years. Basically however his list comprised scrapie; maedi, which is also a disease of sheep but involving the lungs as well as the central nervous system; and a number of tumour viruses such as those concerned in the development of mouse mammary

carcinoma and avian and murine lymphomatosis.    Sigurdsson
recognised that his criteria might require modification in
the light of future knowledge, and, as will be seen later
it seems clear that his original list must also be amended.

Since this initial description, the terms 'slow virus
infection' and 'slow virus disease' have been used to
describe a wide range of conditions, many of which are
obviously not caused by 'slow viruses'.    Because of its
construction, the term "slow virus disease" can obviously
be interpreted in two ways.    It may mean either a disease
resulting from infection with a slow growing agent which
takes a long time to accumulate a sufficiently high titer
to damage enough cells to cause clinical symptoms, or a
disease resulting from the long term persistence in
tissues of a virus which may have replicated rapidly and
reached peak titer without hours or days of infection, but
which the host has been unable to eradicate.    In the latter
group clinical symptoms may also appear after a long interval, but the underlying pathological changes are usually due
to tissue destruction by virus-antibody complexes rather
than to an increase in the number of virus-infected cells.

Following Sigurdsson's initial description there has
been an increasing tendency to group together the clinical
syndromes resulting from both the above processes under the
heading of "slow virus diseases".    In fact, since we began
to write this monograph, at least two separate volumes
entitled "Slow Virus Diseases" have appeared (49, 80) in
which disease processes resulting from slow growing and
persistent viruses are considered together almost without
discrimination.    A typical example has been the inclusion
of the pathological changes occurring in mice a comparatively
long time after infection with Riley (lactate dehydrogenase

elevating) virus.   As has already been said this is one of
the most rapidly replicating viruses known.   However, once
the phase of rapid replication and subsequent decline in
plasma titer has occurred the virus does not disappear, but
stabilises at a level of about $10^6$ infective units/ml -
which is in fact still relatively high - and remains at this
level for the lifetime of the animal.   During this period,
slow degenerative changes can be detected in the lymphoreticular system and renal glomeruli, but except in rare
instances, the animals show no clinical symptoms and little
or no reduction in life span.

It has even been proposed that the sequelae resulting
from specific cellular destruction caused by an acute "fast"
virus infection falls into the category of "slow virus
diseases".   An example of this type of disease is the
suggestion that diabetes mellitus in man may result from
EMC virus infection of the pancreas.   In this case it is
postulated that EMC virus may, as a result of an acute
(short term) infection, destroy the β cells of the pancreas
and leave the patient with this long term, chronic disability.
Not only is the initial infection short lived, but there
seems no necessity even for the long term persistence of the
causative agent.

We recognise that if one begins from the standpoint of
slow virus diseases, it may seem natural to bring together
all slow developing or chronic pathological changes resulting in any way from the initial viral infection.   However
not only do we feel that this diverts attention from differences between the underlying mechanisms of disease production
in the two types of infection but also that if one begins
from the standpoint of 'slow (growing) viruses' it is quite
impossible to include 'fast growing viruses' under the

same heading just because infection with them may result in pathological changes after a relatively long time interval. Consequently it seems necessary to define clearly what we believe the terms 'slow virus', 'slow virus infection' and 'slow virus disease' should mean.

The term 'virus infection' is self explanatory, and 'virus disease' may be defined as a disease resulting from virus infection. These two terms tend to be used inter- changeably, but it is necessary to retain both because infection with a virus does not necessarily result in a recognisable disease. Further the term 'virus infection' does, in general, imply that virus replication takes place (but see latent viruses). The terms 'slow virus infection' and 'slow virus disease' may be defined similarly, but with a 'slow (growing) virus' as the causative agent. In practice there are no known instances of an active slow virus infection not resulting in a slow virus disease but the possibility must not be forgotten, particularly if the terms are to be used interchangeably. Because of the confusion which obviously exists, 'slow viruses' must also be defined in a way which differentiates them from 'latent', 'persistent' and 'temperate' viruses and this necessitates revision of Sigurdsson's original criteria. Some points of difference between these groups have already been made, but the matter is so important that they will be restated as necessary.

A latent virus may be defined as one which is main- tained inside a cell without the production of new infectious virus. Consequently, in this case, virus infection is not necessarily associated with virus replication. However it is possible, and in some cases probable, that maintenance

replication of the nucleic acid or nucleoprotein continues,
and particularly this seems to occur in step with cell
division.   Latent states are usually stable and may persist
for many years, but changes in the state of the host can
disrupt the balance between virus and cell.   When this
occurs the virus may be activated and produce new infectious
virus resulting in the development of clinical disease.
The most common examples are herpes simplex and zoster
viruses which produce typical acute diseases after activation.
However, under certain circumstances a normally rapid virus
may go 'latent' in an altered form.   In such a case,
reactivation may result in the occurrence of what is
apparently a slow virus infection.

The terms 'temperate' and 'persistent' have in practice,
been used indiscriminately for the same group of viruses.
Consequently only the term 'persistent' will be used in this
volume since it accurately describes the type of infection
produced.   Thus the principal feature of 'persistence' is
the continued production of infectious virus (possibly at
reduced levels) in the tissues of the host animal for very
long periods of time - and sometimes indeed for its entire
lifespan.   This persistent infection may have little or no
adverse effect on the health of the animal and, in tissue
cultures, individual cells can continue to produce infectious
virus while retaining their normal cellular functions.

Slow viruses obviously exhibit some of the characteristics of both latent and persistent viruses.   We believe
however that if the terms 'slow virus' and 'slow virus
disease' are to be meaningful they must be defined in the
following way in order to differentiate them from the other
two groups.   The evidence for some of the statements made
will be given later.

1)  A slow virus is one which has a long incubation period.  The upper and lower limits are not easy to define, but bearing in mind the enormous preponderance of virus incubation periods which are less than one month in duration (Fig. 1), an arbitrary requirement of at least three months for the minimum incubation period in man or larger animals seems reasonable.  Most slow virus diseases have a far longer incubation period which as we have indicated, theoretically at least could exceed the life-span of the host, and indeed there is some recent experimental evidence to support this (24).

2)  As in the case of normal viruses, the incubation period of a slow virus may be divided into 'latent' and 'replicative' phases.  A slow virus has both a long latent phase and a slow replication rate.

3)  Although the replication rate is slow, it must be sufficiently rapid to produce a progressive increase in the quantity of virus in the infected organ.

4)  The increase in titer is usually accompanied by a chronic progressive disease which in practice is always severe and usually fatal.

These criteria differentiate slow viruses from those latent viruses in which activation is followed by rapid viral replication and an acute disease.  Some viruses - rabies for example - may have a moderately long latent period due to the time taken for the virus to travel from the site of infection to the site of replication - such as from the extremities to the brain.  Arrival of the virus at the replication site may then be followed by rapid replication and an acute illness.  We feel that special cases of this nature must also be excluded from the slow virus group.

Tumor viruses, which formed a major part of Sigurdsson's original list, must also be excluded.  The increase in our knowledge of these agents, which has accrued since Sigurdsson's day, makes it clear that they came into a special category.  This will be discussed in more detail later.

As the definition of a slow virus relies very heavily on the clinical-pathological effects produced in the intact host we shall attempt to relate the properties of these viruses to the unusual disease processes for which they are responsible.  Indeed, most studies of the slow viruses are perforce associated with the diseases they produce and we must therefore examine this aspect of the problem in some detail.  However, before doing so we will consider some basic first principles which are relevant to virus replication in general.

Table 1
Slow Virus Diseases

| Disease | Primary host | Nucleic acid | Tissue involved | Duration | Outcome |
|---|---|---|---|---|---|
| Kuru*** | Man | ? | CNS | 3-6 years | Fatal |
| Creutzfeldt-Jakob*** | Man | ? | CNS | About 1 yr | Fatal |
| Transmissable mink encephalopathy (TME)*** | Mink | ? | CNS | 6-12 months | Fatal |
| Scrapie*** | Sheep | DNA ? | CNS | 1-3 years | Fatal |
| Progressive multifocal leucoencephalopathy (PML) | Man | DNA | CNS | *8-20 months | Fatal |
| Subacute sclerosing pan-encephalitis (SSPE) | Man | RNA (measles) | CNS | *3-36 months | Fatal |
| Visna-maedi encephalitis or pneumonia | Sheep | RNA** | CNS / Lung | 3-24 months | Fatal / Fatal |
| Serum hepatitis or Australia antigen associated hepatitis | Man | ? | Liver | 1-7 months or chronic | Recovery / Fatal |

* From onset of symptoms;     ** (+ reverse transcriptase);     *** spongiform encephalopathy group

Table 2

Slow diseases in man of possible virus etiology.

| Disease | Tissue involved |
| --- | --- |
| Multiple sclerosis | CNS |
| Schilders disease | CNS |
| Devic's disease | CNS |
| Amyotrophic lateral sclerosis* | CNS |
| Progressive muscular atrophy* | CNS |
| Chronic bulbar paralysis* | CNS |
| Parkinsonian dementia | CNS |
| Paralysis agitans (Parkinson's disease) | CNS |
| Alzheimer's disease | CNS |
| Pick's disease | CNS |
| Chronic polymyositis | Muscle |

* Motor Neuron Disease

CHAPTER III

RATE-GOVERNING STEPS

SOME ASPECTS OF RATE-GOVERNING STEPS IN VIRAL
REPLICATION

We have already indicated that comparatively little
attention seems to have been given to the factors which
govern the rate of viral replication, and in particular to
the reasons why different viruses replicate at such different
rates. If 'fast viruses' and 'slow viruses' are compared
the example already cited (Riley virus vs. scrapie agent)
indicates that in the same animal (mouse) the difference in
replication rate between fast and slow viruses is of the
order of 300:1. Between mouse Riley and sheep scrapie it
approximates to 1000:1, and in man the difference between
influenza and Kuru could be as large as 1500:1. Further,
by far the greatest amount of work to date has been devoted
to fast, or relatively fast, viruses - largely because, as
will become clear, they are by far the easiest group to
study. It therefore seemed to us logical, and indeed
necessary, to begin any enquiry into the nature of slow
viruses and the reasons for their slow growth rate, by

attempting to extrapolate from the information which has
accumulated during studies on fast viruses.    In the absence
of any obvious guide lines indicating reasons for slow
replication we have felt it necessary to go back to first
principles and try to consider as many as we could of the
large number of rate governing factors which appear to be
involved in viral replication to see whether any of them
might cause slow growth under the right conditions.
Clearly it has not been possible in this small volume to
deal with the subject in depth, or even to cover all possible
aspects.    We have therefore necessarily exercised some
selection in considering those factors we consider most
relevant.    Our final conclusions are based as much as
anything on the elimination of mechanisms which seem less
likely to be able to retard viral replication to the extent
necessary to encompass the growth rate of slow viruses.

This chapter will be devoted therefore to:

a)    Factors governing the rate of synthesis of viral macro-
      molecules;  and in particular to the differences
      between synthetic rates of RNA and DNA.

b)    Rates of synthesis of macromolecules in normal tissues
      including as extremes neoplastic and fetal tissues and
      stable tissues such as those of the adult CNS.

c)    Potential rate governing aspects of viral assembly, and
      virus host cell relationships, with particular reference
      to the ability of viruses to 'take over' and direct the
      synthetic machinery of their host cells.

Firstly it must be underlined that the rate of production of all viral components will be governed not only by
those factors which affect the rate of net synthesis of
macromolecules, but also by the ability of the virus to

subvert the rate-governing steps for its own purposes.    So
far as is known all viruses contain a nucleic acid core which
consists of either DNA or RNA which is enclosed within and
protected by a capsid made up of symmetrically arranged
protein molecules.    This nucleocapsid may remain naked or
be enveloped in an outer coat which, while also containing
protein, is usually rich in lipid and carbohydrate.

It is generally accepted that viral agents follow the
central dogma of molecular biology, i.e. that the nucleic
acid core carries the informational requirements for the
synthesis of the complete virus particles (or virions)
together with at least some capacity to organise the infected
cell for the production of the necessary macromolecules.
The basic experimental evidence for this conclusion is that
nucleic acid isolated from a number of DNA and RNA viruses
is itself infective and capable of organising the production
of new complete infectious virions in the host cells.    The
evidence seems reasonably clear cut, although it must always
be borne in mind that, in practice, it is almost impossible
to isolate nucleic acid free from some contamination with
protein or carbohydrate.    Since the infectivity of
isolated nucleic acid is usually very low, i.e. a large
number of nucleic acid molecules are necessary to produce an
infective dose, there is always the possibility that the
infection results from a few nucleic acid molecules
associated with a more than average contamination with
protein.

However it must also be said that the concept that
nucleic acid is essential has not gone unchallenged.    The
suggestion has been made that some viruses - notably the
infective agent of scrapie - do not contain nucleic acid

and therefore must have an informational self-replicating
core consisting of other material such as protein or carbohydrate.   This problem will be dealt with when the nature
of the scrapie agent is discussed later under a separate
heading.

    Before considering possible rate limiting steps in the
synthesis of specific viral nucleic acid, it will first be
relevant to consider briefly some points relating to the
mechanisms involved in the replication of normal cellular
DNA and RNA.   In general, nucleic acids are built up from
cellular pools of the purine and pyrimidine ribo- and
deoxyribo-nucleotides.   These precursors are synthesised
de novo from small molecules and part of any excess is
released into circulation, either as free bases or possibly
nucleosides.   Such preformed bases may be taken up by
other tissues to supplement their own synthetic pathways.
Most tissues in fact are able to make use of both sources
and to switch from one to the other as and when the need
arises.   Except in special circumstances such as rapid cell
division, or perhaps in the terminal stages of infection
with a lytic virus, the supply of these materials is unlikely
to be rate-limiting for the synthesis of either cellular or
viral RNA.   Although similar general principles apply, the
synthesis of DNA precursors is perhaps more complex than
that of RNA, because of the additional pathways necessary
to produce thymidylic acid.   Essentially those involve the
enzymes thymidine kinase and thymidylate synthetase.   In
tissues with a low basic rate of DNA synthesis, the sizes
of the thymidylic acid precursor pools tend to be very
small and the activities of these enzyme systems correspond-
ingly low.   Therefore, in some circumstances the amount of

thymidylic acid available and the mechanisms for producing
it might be rate limiting for DNA synthesis, although this
seems unlikely to be the cause of the low replication rate
of slow viruses.

The precise mechanism by which DNA is actually assembled
in normal cells is still very obscure - and this applies
particularly to mammalian cells.   It seems unlikely that a
single 'DNA polymerase' enzyme exists which is capable of
replicating double stranded DNA unaided, and the complexity
and obscurity of the overall reactions involved is made
clear in recent reviews (33, 44, 52).   The details cannot
possibly be encompassed in this module, but as a general
point it may be said that the proposition has been made that
DNA strand growth occurs by a discontinuous mechanism in
which relatively short daughter strands are produced and
subsequently linked together by ligase enzymes.   These
subsidiary strands are referred to as the 'Okazaki' fragments
after Okazaki and co-workers (66).

Normal cellular RNA synthesis occurs by the linking
together of ribonucleotides on DNA templates.   This
'transcription' process uses the enzyme DNA-dependent RNA
polymerase which binds to the DNA and, after separating the
DNA strands at specific sites, moves along the DNA using one
of the strands as a template to direct the polymerisation of
the ribonucleotides into complementary RNA molecules.   The
process and its control are better understood than that of
the DNA system, but are nevertheless complex, and most of
the information currently available is derived from
bacterial rather than mammalian systems.   In these it has
been suggested that sub units of the RNA polymerase
enzymes (Sigma factors) confer specificity on the replication

process by permitting only certain sites on DNA molecules to
be recognised for the purpose of transcription.   However it
should perhaps be stated that more recent data suggest that
the role of sigma factors may not be so clear cut as was
originally believed.   There are also other protein factors,
which are capable of stimulating the rate of transcription
at certain sites.   In fact the whole process seems highly
regulated and the transcription of specific RNA's can be
switched on and off as necessary.   Despite what may be a
multiplicity of controlling factors it is nevertheless a
matter of experimental evidence that RNA is synthesised at a
rapid rate in most, if not all, mammalian tissues.   This is
especially true of nuclear RNA and, as will be seen in the
next section, is in striking contrast to DNA synthesis,
particularly in stable adult tissue.   Where - as in adult
tissues - there may be little or no net synthesis of RNA,
the rapid rate of production must be balanced by an equally
rate of degradation, although the functional significance of
this overall process is obscure.   Certainly all tissues
abound in nuclease enzymes which, in vitro, can be shown to
degrade RNA very rapidly and most probably they perform this
same function in vivo.   The relationship between RNA
degradation and the more specific regulators of RNA synthesis
in the control of the net synthetic rate, is not clear.
Possibly  the degradative reactions are used to control the
overall rate, while the other regulators are concerned with
the relative amounts of individual, specific RNA's.

    In contrast, cells and tissues appear to vary markedly
in their ability to produce new DNA.   At one end of the
scale are reticulo-endothelial, fetal and certain neoplastic
cells, which have the high rate of DNA synthesis necessary

to support rapid multiplication, and at the other are the
stable adult tissues as a whole.    Although surprisingly
little work has been done on DNA synthesis in such adult
tissues, it is clear that it proceeds at a low to almost
indeterminable rate.    In adult rat central nervous system
(CNS) tissues, for example, the rate of incorporation of
radioactively labelled precursors into DNA is so slow that
the small incorporation which does take place may be due to
the repair of existing DNA, rather than to any net synthesis.
Indeed the mammalian CNS begins to lose cells and its total
DNA content begins to decrease, comparatively early in adult
life.    In rat CNS there is a clear net synthesis and
increase in the cerebral content of DNA up to about four
weeks of age, followed by a slow decrease.    Despite this
the tissues of the CNS support a relatively high rate of
nuclear RNA synthesis at least into adult life (1, 3).
There is no good reason to doubt that a similar situation -
with of course the appropriate time scale - exists in other
species, including man.

Despite a low resting rate of DNA synthesis most adult
tissues exhibit a greater or lesser tendency to regenerate
after injury or resection, so that they still retain the
ability to return to a phase where DNA is rapidly synthesized.
Once again, however, the tissues of the CNS lie at the bottom
of the scale, and show very little regenerative capacity.
It has been said that the glial cells in the CNS (which is
made up of glial and neuronal cells in approximately equal
proportions) do retain some capacity for regeneration, but
this seems to be very limited.    Further, regenerating
tissue obviously requires the production of new RNA and
protein, on what may easily be a massive scale, to keep pace

with the rapid cell division.   Thus in those adult
mammalian tissues which are capable of regeneration, the
balance between synthesis and degradation of RNA can be
altered quickly in the direction of rapid net synthesis.
However, it may perhaps be emphasised here that the overall
control of the various cellular mechanisms involved almost
certainly rests with DNA rather than with RNA itself.

Since all tissues also contain enzymes capable of
degrading DNA it might reasonably be assumed that their
activity will also have to be taken into account when
considering the net synthesis of DNA.   However, in practice,
cellular DNA appears to be protected against, or inaccessible
to them.   In contrast to RNA then, the lack of net synthesis
of DNA in stable adult tissues is due primarily to the very
low synthetic rate.

Now, the essential difference between the pattern of
DNA synthesis in normal and in neoplastic cells lies not so
much in the rate at which it takes place, but in its overall
control and regulation.   Under conditions of rapid synthesis
in reticulo-endothelial, fetal and regenerating normal
tissue, the process is regulated in the interests of the
organism as a whole.   For example, after partial removal of
the liver, growth and DNA synthesis begin rapidly but reduce
to the normal slow rate as the mass of the new liver tissue
approaches that of the original liver.   We have little
knowledge of the control mechanisms which bring this about,
but no doubt both intra- and extra-cellular factors are
involved.   It seems an inescapable conclusion that one of
the essential differences in neoplastic growth is the
inability of the host cells, or the host as a whole, to
regulate and restrain the extent of growth and DNA synthesis.

It is important, however, to emphasise that this inability
does not mean that the unrestrained growth and DNA synthesis
is necessarily rapid.   Tumor growth may be very rapid -
although in general not more rapid than that of fetal or
regenerating tissue - or very slow.   Some human tumors for
example, may take years to reach an appreciable size.   Again,
the mechanisms governing the relevant rates of growth and
DNA synthesis are obscure, but there seem in summary to be
two important points, which will be considered later, in the
context of virus replication.

  1)   DNA synthesis is uncontrolled in neoplastic tissue
in the sense that the mechanisms which would normally halt
it are ineffective.   However, although the rate at which
DNA synthesis proceeds may vary very widely from tumor to
tumor, broadly speaking in each type it is kept relatively
constant.   This must, presumably, mean that some relatively
constant degree of rate control is still operating.

  2)   Again, broadly speaking, the rate controlling
factors - of whatever nature - seem able to exert this
relatively constant influence for long and even very long
periods.   In practical terms therefore a slow, steady,
progressive rate of growth and DNA synthesis can be achieved.

  At this point there is little to be said concerning
cellular protein synthesis except a reminder that the
sequence of amino acids is specified by the triplet code
carried by 'informational' RNA (now almost universally
referred to as messenger (m) RNA), which is expressed through
the association of such RNA with one or more ribosomes.
The same principle applies to the production of virus-specific
proteins, although the details are more complex as will be
seen in the next section.   Protein synthesis in all cells

usually takes place at a relatively rapid rate and seems
unlikely to be a major factor in limiting the rate of virion
production.

Viral DNA, RNA and protein synthesis

In view of the gaps in our present knowledge of the
details of DNA replication in mammalian cells, it is not
possible to say very much more about the mechanisms involved
in the replication of viral double-stranded (ds) DNA.
Most DNA viruses appear to utilise host DNA polymerising
systems, and it has been suggested that, like cellular DNA,
the DNA of SV 40 and polyoma viruses at least are made by
the two stage process of linking polynucleotide fragments
together (38).

Although similar in principle, the mechanism of replication of viral RNA is more complicated than that of
cellular RNA because there are three categories of viral
RNA:

1) double-stranded (ds) consisting of a combination of an
   mRNA strand and a vegetative (v) RNA strand,

2) single-stranded (ss) RNA of either the 'm' or 'v' type.
Normally 'v' type RNA must be transcribed to 'm' type RNA in
order to be translated into specific viral proteins.
Further, since RNA-directed nucleic acid polymerase systems
have not been demonstrated in uninfected cells, the viral
RNA must carry its own transcriptase(s).   The details of
all the mechanisms involved in viral RNA replication cannot
be given in this volume for reasons of space and the interested reader is directed to "The Biology of Animal Viruses"
(second edition) (39).   Despite the complexity of some of
these mechanisms, there seems no obvious reason why the
synthesis of viral RNA should not proceed rapidly and at the

limit to which the synthetic machinery is capable.

One very interesting problem which arises is how, as seems to be the case, viral transcriptase replicates viral rather than host RNA.   However, since this aspect has been lucidly discussed by Spiegelman (76) it will not be further considered here.

To summarise, not only does the synthesis of viral RNA seem geared to rapidity, as is cellular RNA but there is no clear evidence to suggest how it might be reduced by the very large factor which would be required for a slow virus.

So far as DNA viruses are concerned, some at least carry a DNA directed RNA polymerase enzyme within their virions (53), and this should facilitate the rapid synthesis of the necessary mRNA.   Although the absence of such an enzyme could theoretically slow down the early stages in the replication of a virus, in practice there is little evidence that this is a major factor.

In comparison with cellular protein synthesis viral protein synthesis is more complex because of the variability of the messenger RNA produced by different viruses.   Viral mRNA may be either monocistronic or polycistronic.   Mono-cistronic messengers are translated all at one time into a 'giant' protein which is subsequently cleaved at specific points to form a number of smaller proteins.   A poly-cistronic messenger is a single long strand, but containing a number of initiation and termination points, so that the whole is not transcribed at once.

Alternatively the genome may be segmented (reovirus and influenza virus for example) in which case mRNA's are transcribed individually from each segment.

One essential difference between mono- and polycistronic viral messengers is that in the former case equal amounts of all the virus-specific proteins are made at the same time. The synthesis of proteins individually under the influence of polycistronic messengers allows control to be exerted at the translation level, on the amounts of each protein synthesised. In at least a proportion of viruses (phage for example) some of the proteins produced are able to govern the synthetic rate of others. However the purpose of this seems more likely to ensure that the individual proteins are produced at the correct rates in the interests of the overall process of phage assembly, than to be rate limiting. Consequently, taking viral protein synthesis as a whole, it is difficult to see any reason why one individual step should be severely rate limiting. All that can be said is that if for any reason one essential protein were to be made in insufficient quantities, the production of infectious virions would obviously proceed at a reduced rate. Further, that in such circumstances the proportion of incomplete and non-infectious virions would increase.

## VIRUS-HOST CELL RELATIONSHIPS

The previous section has not produced any obvious clues to the identity of the factors which must govern the slow, controlled replication rate of slow viruses. However, it has been noted that normal DNA synthesis can obviously take place at very widely different rates. In this section it is proposed to extend the enquiry to the possible rate governing factors which may arise from the interaction of viruses with their host cells.

In order to do this let us begin by summarising briefly
the events which take place in bacterial cells after infection with a lytic virus.   Once the virus has penetrated the
cell wall and the uncoating process has occurred, the bare
nucleic acid finds itself in a very unfriendly, if not active-
ly hostile environment.   Subsequent events will then be
determined largely by the ability of the nucleic acid core
to survive, and at the same time to compete with, and direct
the synthetic mechanisms of the infected cell, while over-
coming any attempts it may make to resist.   Some viral
nucleic acids, which might be considered as being the most
"successful", are able to subvert cellular systems almost
completely to the production of new viral nucleic acid,
together with the necessary structural proteins.   Under
these circumstances the infected cell becomes little more
than a factory for the manufacture of new virus, and when it
becomes packed with virus particles, the cell membrane
disintegrates, liberating the contents to infect other cells.
This "lytic" phenomenon is less common, and probably of less
importance, than used to be thought, but nevertheless the
whole process illustrates the potential some viruses have for
rapid, efficient and superbly organised 'take over' of the
cells they infect.   In summary this may be described as the
basic strategy of a fast virus.

Shortly after infection with a fast RNA virus there is
a rapid reduction in the rate of synthesis of host cell protein and RNA.   The extent to which this occurs is very
variable.   When Hela cells are infected with poliovirus,
for example, their protein synthetic rate begins to decrease
almost immediately and falls rapidly to below 10% of normal
after six hours.   On the contrary the synthesis of virus

specific protein begins slowly and reaches a peak three
hours after infection.   Other viruses do not produce such a
dramatic effect and host protein synthesis is limited only
to around 50% of its normal rate.   It seems clear that apart
from variability inherent in the nature of the viruses
themselves (ability to subvert the normal host cell machinery
for example) the results will depend on whether the infection
is in cells in culture or in vivo.   The degree of inhibition
must also depend on whether the virus is of the lytic type
by which the host cell is rapidly killed and the virus
released or whether, in order to proceed by slower growth
and budding, it is necessary for the virus to hold the host
cell in a captive but viable state for a longer period.

   Broadly speaking the effects of infection on host cell
protein synthesis seem to be mediated by the production of
a factor or factors, probably of a protein nature, which
are not normally present in the cell.   Such factors may be
carried within the virion, or translated from viral mRNA.
They inhibit the transcription of host cell RNA including of
course host messenger, possibly by combining with and
masking part of the host DNA templates.   Cellular protein
synthesis also appears to be affected by a disaggregation
of polysomes, which is not associated with the inhibition of
host RNA synthesis.   Even where cellular messenger is still
in the arena (and in mammalian cells many messengers have
a comparatively long half life) it seems unable to bind in
stable fashion with ribosomes, unlike segments of the viral
RNA.   In some way then its competitive ability appears to
be impaired.   Normal DNA synthesis is also decreased in
these infected cells and may cease altogether.   Since, of
course, the bulk of DNA synthesis is synchronously related

to cell division, any inhibition resulting from virus infection may not be due to a direct effect on the synthetic
mechanisms themselves.   Similar effects can be brought
about simply by a sufficient inhibition of RNA and protein
synthesis produced in other ways.

Infection with DNA viruses such as vaccinia and herpes
simplex also results in an inhibition of RNA and protein
synthesis in host cells, but the effects seem to be much
less clear cut than those just described.   Some evidence in
fact, suggests that infection with the DNA viruses polyoma
and SV40 may actually initiate a round of DNA synthesis and
cell division.   However, 'take over' of the cell is an
important feature associated with infection with DNA viruses,
and one significant aspect of this may be illustrated by
considering the infection of E.coli with phages of the T-even
series.   In this case the DNA of the infective agent contains
the abnormal pyrimidine base 5 -hydroxymethylcytosine and
this largely replaces cytosine which is, of course, the
normal base.   Obviously then, unless the new hydroxymethyl-
ated base can be produced, viral replication cannot take
place.   In fact, after infection and concomitantly with the
associated inhibition of their normal nucleic acid and protein synthesis, the host cells are programmed to synthesise
a new hydroxymethylase enzyme able to convert cytosine to
the required 5-hydroxymethyl derivative.

There would seem to be two ways in which the synthesis
of new enzymes can be achieved as a result of virus infection.
Either a segment of the viral DNA must serve directly as a
template to specify the new protein or indirectly via the
transcription of a new messenger RNA.   There have been
reports of direct transcription of protein from DNA, but

there is so far no evidence that this occurs in viral systems.
Consequently the latter alternative, i.e. via RNA, seems most
probable, and indeed has been shown experimentally for
vaccinia and other DNA viruses.   It is of interest to note
the similarity between the properties of messenger RNA
produced in this way, and those already mentioned for viral
RNA acting as messenger.   In both cases, the evidence
suggests that, in some way, viral messenger has a facility
for combining with host polysomes or ribosomes which is
denied to normal host messengers after infection has taken
place.

Thus virus-infected cells cannot only be programmed to
produce new 'replicase'  enzymes to make viral RNA (and in
some circumstances viral DNA) but also to make new enzymes
for the production of new precursors where the viral
nucleic acid differs fundamentally in composition from that
of the host.   However, since the known examples in which
these changes occur are associated with fast acting agents,
the necessity to make such enzymes does not seem to be a
potential 'slowing' factor - at least not when considered
in relation to the time scale of 'slow' viruses.  Presumably
this is because the viruses in question carry enough coding
information, either to specify the new enzymes completely or
to bring about appropriate modifications of existing host
enzymes.   There seems no obvious reason why such new
enzymes would not be rapidly produced, particularly where,
as part of the overall process, the virus has interfered
with the synthesis by the host of its own RNA and protein.

There is a further spectrum of both DNA and RNA viruses
which do not seem to be quite so successful in 'taking over'
their host cells, and consequently must exist in a rather

more symbiotic relationship with them.   In many such cases
the amount of viral nucleic acid produced may be only a very
small proportion of the total - particularly in the case of
RNA viruses, or DNA viruses in dividing cells.   It may
perhaps be stressed here that there seems to be no obvious or
clear division between this group and the 'take-over' group
of viruses.   However, it does seem reasonable to suppose
that the less the 'take over' ability, the more the virus
will find itself in the position of having to compete on
more equal, or even unequal, terms with its host cell.   It
also seems obvious that such a situation is likely to result
in an overall slowing of the rate of virus replication.
What is not clear is how far viruses of this type need, or
are even able, to specify new enzymes of the types discussed
above.   Since the production of new, specific enzymes may
well be an important factor in 'take over', it might be
suggested that the 'symbiotic' group of viruses are able
either to make use of host enzymes directly or after
only minor modifications.   Possibly, if it were necessary
to stimulate the production of an existing host enzymes
normally present in very small quantities to meet the new
demands, such a process might proceed comparatively slowly,
particularly in adult mammalian cells.


THE VIRAL COAT.   Although the viral nucleic acid core
carries the replicative capacity, the capsid protein and
where present, the envelope also have important roles to
play in the production and properties of the complete virion.
The outermost layer of the virion, whether it be capsid or
envelope, is necessary for its entry into the cell.   In the
case of some viruses it is possible to infect cells with

nucleic acid extracted from purified virions or virus infected cells, but there is no evidence that this is anything
other than a laboratory exercise.    Initial contact between
virion and host cell results from Brownian motion and may be
followed by more or less stable attachment.    The sites of
attachment on the surface of the host cell have a topography
which matches the outer layer of the virion and binds it by
electrostatic forces.    No doubt the closeness of fit will
be a factor influencing the ease of entry, and therefore the
ability of a virus to infect one tissue and not another.
The bound virion is drawn into the (non-bacterial) cell by
phagocytosis (or viropexis) - which is most easily observed
in tissue cultures, but in the intact host the mechanisms of
entry into individual cells appear to be very similar.
However, since the whole process of the penetration of
animal viruses into cells has been extensively reviewed by
Dales (20) it will not be further considered here.

The necessity for the production of these specific coat
proteins along with viral nucleic acid has already been
mentioned, and clearly complete new infective virions could
not be formed without them.    These proteins are specified
by viral messenger RNA and will be synthesised automatically
so long as the relevant host mechanisms are left intact.
These should in fact be usable without any major modifications
being necessary, since, so far as is known, there is little
or no inherent specificity in the process apart from the
messenger RNA.    It is clear then why host protein synthesis
is not immediately and completely inhibited - even after
infection by the most efficient take-over virus.   Not only
must the synthesis of the viral coat proteins be allowed to
proceed, but it must proceed at an accelerated rate if it is

to keep pace with viral nucleic acid production.   Further,
the large number of enzymes and accessory factors necessary
to keep the host's synthetic machinery operating must be
maintained in adequate amounts.   Even the production of
adenosine and guanosine triphosphates, which are essential
for protein synthesis, requires the integrity of the anaero-
bic glycolysis pathways, and for full efficiency, those of
the Krebs cycle as well.   However, as has been pointed out,
where a virus replicates so rapidly that it is liberated,
and its host cell is dead, within a few hours, the host
synthetic machinery has only to be maintained in an operative
condition for a short time.

The problem of how viral messenger is able to oust
cellular messenger, or render it ineffective, has already
been posed.   However, it seems that we must also ask "By
what mechanism can the virus also select and preserve that
part of the host cell machinery required by it, while
suppressing the rest"?   The only logical answer would seem
to be that cellular systems must be broadly divisible into
two groups - those which control, and those which are con-
tolled, and a successful virus is able to slot itself into
and override the first group.

The capsid proteins, being in most immediate contact
with the core, are probably of special importance and,
consequently, at an early stage in the infective process
viral nucleic acid must be diverted from the self-replication
process to act as, or to transcribe, messenger RNA able to
specify them.   Measurements in the case of encephalomyo-
carditis virus have indicated the closely coupled nature of
the synthesis of core, capsid and complete virions.   In
infected mouse ascites cells, in which a very rapid produc-

tion occurs, the viral RNA core is made during the 3-7 hour
period after infection, and the capsid proteins follow a
similar course at an equally rapid rate, but with a delay of
about an hour.   Complete virus (in this case RNA + capsid)
seems to be produced almost as soon as the capsid is formed,
and the importance of such a rapid association of viral
components will be discussed subsequently.


RATE LIMITATION OF VIRAL REPLICATION.   At this point we may
perhaps remind ourselves, that, in chemical terms, when an
end product is the result of a sequence of reactions the
overall rate at which the whole process can proceed is
governed by the rate of the slowest reaction.   Beginning
with nucleotides and amino acids as precursors, the same
principle must apply to the production of new, complete
virions.   However, not only are virions multi-component
systems, in which each component is constructed by a sequence
of reactions which are, to at least some extent, unique, but
the components themselves must also be brought together and
assembled into the final complex.   It also seems reasonable
to assume that unless specific regulatory factors intervene,
new virions will be produced as fast as the synthetic
reactions and assembly processes permit.   Further, when the
host is an intact animal, the new virions must spread to and
infect other cells in a continuous cycle to build up the
virus titer in the tissue as a whole.
    Many aspects of the processes involved in the assembly
of new virions have been touched on already.   However, in
order to emphasise the complexity of the complete sequence
in a host animal it may be of value to summarise the events
which occur during an infective  process, beginning from the

instant when the first virion presents itself at the first
cell membrane.    Comments will also be made on the probable
extent to which the various steps might be rate limiting so
far as the overall process is concerned.

The sequence may be conveniently divided into six
stages.

Stage 1.   Entry of virus to cells.    This is of course a
prerequisite for infection and replication and if it does
not occur the virus can proceed no further.    It may be
worth pointing out here that different tissues in the same
animal host may vary widely in their susceptibility to virus
attachment and subsequent entry.    However the overall effect
on incubation period arising from difficult as against easy
entry is likely to do little more than parallel the increase
which results from a reduction in the number of infectious
particles in the inoculum.    This phenomenon happens with all
viruses, and even with scrapie (vide infra), a reduction in
the infective dose from half a million units to just one,
has been found to lengthen the incubation period by a factor
of only two.    Consequently the rate of entry seems unlikely
to be a major factor in determining the rate of virion production.

Stage 2.   Uncoating of the virus.    This process is not
fully understood, but generally speaking, unless it occurs,
the nucleic acid core of the virus will remain masked and
unavailable for copying.    How frequently such a failure of
uncoating occurs is not known, but when it does, either the
degradation of the whole virion, or latency would be the
most probable results.    Uncoating may be delayed for a more

limited period, and this has been demonstrated in tissue
culture.    Cultures of hamster cells infected with polyoma
virus rapidly absorb the virus and it can then be detected
intracellularly by immunofluorescence.    As the cells divide,
the virions may remain in the cytoplasm of the daughter cells
for several generations before being uncoated.    However,
once uncoating has taken place there seems no obvious reason
why an initial delay should have any effect on the subsequent
rate of replication.

In passing, it may be of interest to note that there
appear to be exceptions to the bald statement that a virus
must be uncoated before beginning its replication cycle.
Kates and Beeson  (53)  have reported that vaccinia virus
induces the synthesis of messenger RNA before the uncoating
mechanism has proceeded far enough to release viral DNA from
the core.    This suggests that activity may begin when only
partial uncoating has taken place, but of course such a
process could hardly do other than speed up virion production.


Stage 3.    Replication.    After the uncoating process, the
nucleic acid core enters into the metabolic activity of the
cell in the way already described.    The viral nucleic acid
must act as, or organise the production of messenger RNA for
the synthesis of perhaps several envelope and capsid proteins
and often specific replicase or other enzymes.    It must
organise its own replication, and to a greater or lesser
extent 'take over' or compete with the cell's own synthetic
processes.    Where the virus has an outer envelope as well
as a capsid the necessary lipids and polysaccharides must be
either synthesised de novo or diverted from the host cell's
own production.

Stage 4.   Assembly.   Not only must the programming of the
synthesis of all the necessary components be organised, but
for full efficiency in the production of complete virions the
right amount of each component must be produced, and made
available, in the right place at the right time.   An example
of the close synchrony of the synthesis of RNA and capsid
protein and their assembly into virions has already been
given, but for those who want more detailed information,
there are recent reviews of the topic (15, 36).

Stage 5.   Maturation and Release.   The release of new
virions from infected cells is essential for the spread of
the virus.   A major problem in the study of release is that
many investigations have used monolayer cell cultures which
do not always give a true picture of the events occurring
in the whole animal.   However, it is possible to distinguish
four main patterns of release.   The "burst" phenomenon of
phage, in which the bacterial cell becomes filled with new
particles and then bursts, does not appear to have any
genuine parallels among the viruses of vertebrates.
Probably the commonest method is that of budding by the
larger, enveloped, viruses, in which final maturation and
release occur simultaneously.   In the case of the RNA-
containing viruses (myxo, rhabdo, corona, arena and leukoviruses) the nucleoprotein component is assembled at areas
of the cytoplasmic membrane which have been altered by the
replacement of host cell proteins with virus-specified
material, although the original lipids appear to be retained.
The nucleocapsid is then enclosed with a 'bleb', or bud, of
altered cell membrane which is "nipped" off from the cell
surface to form the new, enveloped, virion.   The DNA-

containing herpes viruses are formed in a similar manner by
budding from the nuclear membrane into channels leading
directly to the intercellular spaces.   The small RNA viruses
(picorna and togaviruses) appear to be assembled (in vivo)
within cytoplasmic structures formed from expanded endo-
plasmic reticulum.   These structures are connected to the
cell surface by tubules through which the new virions are
continuously extruded.   It can be seen that release by
budding or extrusion is a rapid process which commences as
soon as new virions are formed and it is unlikely that this
could be a rate-limiting step.   On the other hand, the
fourth method of release occurs when the mature virions form
crystals in the nucleus of the infected cell (adenoviruses)
or in its cytoplasm (picornaviruses in vitro, reoviruses and
orbiviruses) or are intimately bound to membrane within the
cell (scrapie).   In these cases the death of the cell is
required before new virus is released and, if the infected
cells can survive for a long period, this would be a rate-
limiting step in the overall infection process.

Stage 6.   Spread of infection.   Stages 1-5 take place
essentially within the confines of each of the cells which
were infected when the virus first entered the host.
However, in intact animals this will be only a very small
proportion of the total.   Consequently, for the overall
virus titer to build up enabling it to spread through the
tissues, the new virions produced in the infected cells must
enter and infect new cells, and the whole sequence repeat
itself over and over again.   The complications arising at
this stage - the production of antibodies by the host in an
attempt to destroy the invader, and the resistance to

infection induced in uninfected cells by the appearance of
interferon, will be discussed later.  For the present, these
defense mechanisms are not so much rate-limiting as infection-
aborting in their effect and between them are responsible for
the recovery of the host.  In any event, as will be seen
later, they do not seem to operate to any significant extent
in slow virus infections.  Clearly, then, for a virus to
survive and multiply, a very large number of integrated
sequential steps are involved.  Such a complex process is
obviously associated with many problems which must be overcome
it it is to proceed efficiently.

First let us consider again the rapid degradation of RNA
which accompanies the forward synthetic reactions.  The
enzymes which are assumed to be involved are relatively non-
specific and there is no very good reason to think that viral
RNA, once uncoated, would be resistant to attack.  The same
is true of the new viral RNA made by replication of the
original.  One obvious way of protecting such new naked RNA
would then be to ensure (a) that capsid protein is rapidly
produced, and (b) that it is brought together with the nucleic
acid as quickly as possible.  What can be done in this
respect has already been shown, but the possibilities of
error are obviously large, and any mis-timing of the
replication sequences or the arrival at the rendezvous could
render the infection almost entirely abortive.  Further, it
does not seem clear to what extent the viral RNA is susceptible to enzyme attack while it is actually involved in the
replication process.  It it is, then at least some of the
newly synthesised RNA would have to be fed back to maintain
the synthetic rate.  The capsid protein does, of course,
have the great advantage of stability, at least in comparison

with RNA.   However, it is not entirely clear whether the
intracellular production of such foreign protein may stimulate
the synthesis of enzymes to degrade it - which could reduce
its 'advantage'.   Any such attempt by the cell would, of
course, depend for its success on the cell's ability to
evade the constraints placed upon it by the infecting virus.
These remarks have concentrated on RNA because the probabil-
ities are more clear-cut.   It was said earlier that although
cells also contain enzymes able to degrade DNA, most
cellular DNA appears to be relatively inaccessible.   However,
it seems probable that viral DNA, so long as it remains 'free'
within its host cell, will be subject to the same hazards.

    It is hardly surprising then, that there are variations
in the rates of replication of the spectrum of viruses in
the range of host cells and tissues.   It has been suggested
that the most rapid replication, occurring in the shortest
period after infection would occur with RNA viruses, and
with those which are able to take over their host cells
most effectively.   The less they are able to do this, the
slower will be the rate of production of new virions.
Failure in this respect will also tend to result in the
production of larger proportions of virus particles which
are altered or incomplete in a way which makes them non-
infective.   The same result would also be expected it there
was any hitch in the synthesis of a single component - one
of the capsid proteins for example.

    Despite these problems, it is nevertheless clear that
the production of new virions can - potentially at any rate -
proceed very rapidly and efficiently.   In the example of
Riley virus, it has already been said that up to $10^{12}$ infective doses arise in each ml. of mouse serum within about 16

hours after infection.   For this to be attained, it seems
obvious that all the stages involved must be working at high
efficiency in every aspect.   Further, although such very
fast viruses - indeed like the slow viruses - are in a minority, there are a sufficient number in a sufficient range of
tissues to indicate that this potential for rapid viral
replication is widespread, and the suggestion has already
been made that such rapidity is related to 'take over'
ability.   In the host-virus complex associated with less
successful viruses, normal cellular synthesis takes place to
a greater or lesser extent concomitantly with that of viral
components.   It has already been suggested that new virions
are likely to be produced more slowly in such circumstances.
The most likely reason would seem to be a slowing of one or
more of the processes involved in the replication phase
(Stage 3) due to competition between host and viral systems
restricting the capacity available to the latter.   Can it
then be postulated that a slow virus is one in which this
trend is considerably extrapolated, and if so, that latent
viruses represent the ultimate limit in which host-virus
competition is so weighted against the virus that to all
intents and purposes its replication rate is zero?

    As indicated previously the overall rate of virion
production could be limited by slowing the rate of any one
of the many synthetic reactions - perhaps relating to only
one of the viral components.   In a relatively simple system
such a method of rate control would be possible, even to the
drastic extent which would be required, without necessarily
causing any complications.   However, it is difficult, if not
impossible, to see how this could be achieved in a system as
complex as the production of complete, infectious virions

without losing the overall control and cohesiveness of the
system which seems so essential.  For example, many,
probably insuperable, difficulties would arise if a number
of rapidly produced viral components had to be stockpiled
while waiting for supplies of a component being produced at
such a drastically reduced rate.  For example, nucleic acid
overproduced would either be degraded or stimulate interferon
production in neighbouring cells.

In summary, it is not difficult to see that variations
in the rates of the synthetic reactions and the relative
efficiency of events such as the coming together of core
and capsid protein could, within limits, alter the overall
rate of production of new virions.  However, such processes
are common to all viruses and prima facie would seem most
likely to operate within the period of 4 weeks already
specified as covering the range of incubation periods of the
vast majority of them.  If this view is correct, there seems
no obvious way of sufficiently extending the limits on the
rates of any of these processes to encompass and explain the
controlled 'slowness' of slow viruses and this must be the
tentative answer to the question posed at the beginning of
this general section.  It therefore seems necessary to look
for an additional and essential primary key to the problem,
outside the parameters considered so far.  Possibly the
most significant clue to its nature which has emerged is
the restraint, slowness and control of cellular DNA replication, which has been shown to occur in several situations,
and which, in the case of cell division, is associated with
the control of the net synthesis of the requisite RNA and
protein.  This seems to have obvious analogies with the
slow virus process, and in conjunction with the evidence so

far presented, tentatively suggests that the key to the slow
virus problem lies in the arena of control of DNA replication
and therefore that the nucleic acid core of a slow virus must
be based on DNA rather than RNA.   However, before taking
this line of thought any further, it will be of advantage to
consider the biological and biochemical properties of a
typical slow virus.   Because more work has been done on the
properties of scrapie virus (a member of the spongiform
encephalopathy group - Table 1) than on all the other slow
viruses combined, we shall begin by detailing the early
history of scrapie and continue to the controversy which has
arisen over the nature of the causative agent.

CHAPTER IV


SCRAPIE



Scrapie is a naturally occurring disease of the central nervous system of sheep and goats which has been recognised for perhaps as long as 300 years, although the name 'scrapie' has been in use for only just over 100 years.

In sheep the disease is characterised by an insidious onset associated with behavioural changes such as nervousness and excitability, and physical signs such as tremors, incoordination and lethargy. The symptoms progress over the course of some months to a fatal outcome. In many cases there appears to be an associated cutaneous irritation which leads the sheep to rub themselves raw on any available stump or post. From this latter effect the name 'scrapie' is derived.

Although scrapie is comparatively rare it is nevertheless widespread and probably endemic in many countries. Its

recognition outside Europe seems to have been comparatively
recent, positive diagnoses not being made until about 1939 in
Canada, 1947 in the USA and 1952 in Australia.   The
importation of infected sheep from Britain has been blamed
for this apparent spread of the disease.   However it is by
no means certain that scrapie has not existed unrecognised
in these countries for a much longer period, particularly
since it is now clear that there is a range of scrapie
strains which show variable pathology and clinical symptoms.


EARLY EXPERIMENTS


     In any progressive disease of unknown cause, sooner or
later the question arises 'Is it caused by an infective
transmissable agent?' and, therefore, 'Can it be transmitted
from diseased to healthy animals?'.   The normal way of
attempting this is to inoculate healthy animals by an
appropriate route with tissue preparations taken from diseased
animals in the hope that they in turn will develop the same
disease.   In general it is much easier to transmit infection
to animals of the same species than to cross species barriers,
and as we shall see this causes many problems in attempts to
establish the transmissability of human slow virus diseases.
     In the 1920s there were a number of attempts to transmit
scrapie which were unsuccessful until Cuille and Chelle
realised that other investigators may not have waited a
sufficiently long time for the disease to develop - even
though some of the experiments had continued for as long as
6-9 months.   In 1932 they inoculated 9 sheep, by several
different routes, with spinal cord preparations taken from a
sheep severely affected by scrapie (or 'La tremblant du

mouton'). Seven of these animals died from intercurrent infections or were killed for various reasons before 9 months had elapsed, but the remaining two eventually developed the symptoms of scrapie and died, apparently from that cause. The experiment was repeated with two further sheep. The first of these began to look sick after 14 months, showed definite scrapie symptoms after 16 months and died about 3 months later. The second ran a similar but even slower course, and died just over 2 years after inoculation. The number of animals involved was of course very small, but Cuille and Chelle concluded (17):

1. Scrapie is an infectious, transferable illness.

2. The virus lives in the CNS.

3. The incubation period is about 14-22 months.

In further experiments, the agent was filtered through gauze and a Chamberland L3 filter and inoculated into two 3 month old lambs. Both developed scrapie symptoms after 13 months and died after 16 months. This was the first experiment to give any real indication that a filterable (virus-like) agent was involved, although by modern standards the number of animals was again very small, and little attempt seems to have been made to check the bacterial sterility of the inocula (18). In the last paper of the series Cuille and Chelle (19) failed to transmit scrapie to rabbits, but the disease was successfully transmitted to two goats. The authors drew attention to the fact that the incubation period (25-26 months) was longer than with sheep (usually < 18 months) and that the disease in goats was different - predominantly paralytic with no skin irritation.

The extraordinary thing about their claim was the fact that one to two years had to elapse before the appearance of

disease in the inoculated animals and this led to much
scepticism at the time.    It must also be pointed out that a
single successful transmission of disease from affected to
healthy animals, although highly suggestive, is not acceptable
beyond doubt as proof that the disease is caused by a replicating transmissable factor.    It is just possible, for
example, that if there was some toxic material in the tissues
of the disease animal, then sufficient might be present in
tissue inocula to affect a healthy animal.    However, if this
were the case serial transmission (inoculation from diseased
to healthy→becoming diseased and inoculated to healthy and
so on for several passages) would dilute out any such factor,
and rapidly bring the transmissability to a halt.    The first
person to serially transfer scrapie from sheep to sheep over
at least 9 passages, showing beyond reasonable doubt that a
replicating infective agent was involved, was R. D. Wilson
working at Compton, England in the 1940's.

The length of the incubation period had already shown
that the scrapie 'virus' was extremely unusual and at the time
this fact was sufficient for many to query whether it was
really a virus at all in the accepted sense.    For many
subsequently discovered reasons this question mark has hung
over scrapie right up to the present time.    No other known
virus required anything like this very long time interval
after inoculation to produce disease, and the more its
properties were compared with those of classical viral
agents the more unusual they seemed to become.    It may be
instructive to underline here the formidable difficulties
involved in the early work in carrying out even the simplest
experiments which are normally applied to viruses to test
their properties - ease of inactivation by heat and by such

chemical agents as ether, chloroform and formalin for
example.    To begin with 'slow' viruses had not yet been
recognised.    The investigators, with no guide lines, had
the problem of devising the best experiments to be carried
out in large farm animals in which the only indication of
the presence of virus in any inoculated material was the
development of clinical signs after a prolonged period -
possibly as long as three years.    Even a simple virus
titration was almost an impossibility because of the number
of animals required.    Also, most workers found that about
one inoculated sheep in three never developed the disease at
all due, as we now know, to the influence of genetic factors.
During the early studies the transmission of the disease to
goats was confirmed, and it now seems clear that scrapie also
occurs naturally in this species.    However, here at least,
inoculation was virtually 100% successful.

Nevertheless the early work with large farm animals
served not only to place on a firm footing the suggestion
that the disease was caused by a filterable (virus-like)
transmissable agent but also that the agent had unusual
properties of resistance to heat and the action of chemical
substances compared with most known viruses.    Again it must
be emphasised that all experiments up to the early 1960's
were necessarily perfunctory.    Experiments had to be set up
on an 'all or nothing' basis (i.e. showing either that
infectivity was present or it was not) using a very small
number of animals in each group.    Only in some cases was
any indication obtained of the extent of any reduction in
agent titer, by the introduction of one or two animals
inoculated with intermediate dilutions.    It also began to
be recognised that a lengthened incubation period was able

to give some indication of the extent of any reduction in
virus titer.   A summary of the results obtained in this
early work has been given in a paper by Pattison (69).
Very briefly they show that scrapie infectivity persisted
after:-  boiling for several hours, exposure to 5% chloroform or 2% phenol at $37^{o}$ for 13 days, ether extraction,
several cycles of freezing and thawing, treatment with RNAse
or DNAse.   The presence was reported of active scrapie agent
in louping-ill vaccine containing 0.35% formalin and in
scrapie sheep brain pickled in formalin.


BIOLOGY OF THE SCRAPIE AGENT

     Once the cause of a disease in large animals - or human
beings for that matter - has been established as a transmissable 'virus' it obviously becomes a matter of some
urgency to attempt to infect small laboratory animals with
the disease since these can be studied much more easily.
Only in this way can the laboratory investigation of the
agent be facilitated.   The failures in this respect have
already been mentioned, but in the early 1960's Chandler,
working at the Agricultural Research Council Insitute at
Compton, England, gave a great impetus to scrapie research
by successfully transmitting the disease to mice and rats.
This eased the problem of experimental investigation, but
even in mice the time from infection to death, which is still
the most unequivocal endpoint, occupies between six and
twelve months.   Even a simple virus titration still not only
necessitates tying up large amounts of animal house space
for a prolonged period, but also requires the investigator
to wait all that time for the result of each step.   Small

wonder that the majority of workers in the field of infectious
agents have preferred to deal with the more usual and rapidly
acting viruses.   It is nevertheless true that of the 'slow'
group of agents, scrapie has proved the least difficult to
investigate and despite the results obtained from the more
recent successful transmission of the other agents of the
spongiform encephalopathy group to primates, there is at
present very little option to basing most of our knowledge
of the nature of slow viruses on conclusions derived from
the study of scrapie.   Ironically enough some of the results
obtained have led many investigators to the view that the
infective agent of scrapie does not really fall within the
accepted definition of a virus.   The question which has
arisen is 'Does the scrapie agent contain nucleic acid as
part of its structure?'   If the answer is 'no' then we are
dealing with a hitherto unknown and uncharacterised process
of replication or self-multiplication, and such a conclusion
would raise the further problem of whether any of the other
slow viruses are self-multiplying agents which do not
contain nucleic acid.   If this were so, slow  viruses might
well be removed entirely from the classical virus arena.
It would therefore seem very necessary to consider the
relevant evidence relating to the scrapie agent, and its
interpretation, in some detail in an attempt to resolve this
basic problem.

       In the first place, it is quite clear that if its
slowness is accepted, there is very little biological evidence
that the scrapie agent is not a true virus.   It is clearly
transmissible in the same manner as classical viruses and it
can be titrated by standard procedures.   The results have
shown that after the inoculation of susceptible animals with

a few infective doses, the titer in the brain rises eventually
to at least $10^8$ infective doses/g. wet weight.    In mice,
confirming and extending the original studies with sheep, it
has been demonstrated that this process can be repeated
serially for an indefinite period, which shows beyond doubt
that a true multiplication or self-replication process is
involved.    Scrapie may also be transmitted by intraperitoneal,
or other peripheral routes of infection and Field has shown,
by histological examination, that the way in which scrapie
spreads into the brain after infection at distant sites is
typical of a neurotropic virus.    It is true that, so far,
no structures have been visualised in the electron microscope
which can be unequivocally labelled scrapie agent, although
such claims have been made recently (16, 65).    However, the
presence of the agent can be detected in brain by its cytopathic effects.    Failure to visualise is, of course, by no
means unknown in virus work, and may merely indicate that
the virus is unusually small, or fits unobtrusively into the
background, or both.

There are of course other methods besides direct
visualisation and measurement in the electron microscope
which have commonly been used to determine the size of
viruses and other macromolecules.    One is to pass a suspension of the virus through a series of filters with progressively reducing APD (average pore diameter) and measure the
infectivity of the filtrate at each stage.    For various
reasons, including the presence of any asymmetry in the
particles, such measurements do not give an exact estimate of
the particle sizes, but for general purposes the results
are usually close enough.    Also, centrifugation of suspensions of virus particles may be used to show how fast the

infectivity sediments in comparison with known standard
particles.   Such studies on the scrapie agent have suggested
that infectivity is associated with particles down to about
40nm in diameter - which is typical small virus size.
However, if these 40nm particles were free virions one would
expect to be able to visualise them as such in the electron
microscope.   The failure to do this, and the experimental
observation that large amounts of host cell membrane structures
appear to be associated with the particles carrying scrapie
infectivity, has led to suggestions that the infective
particles consist of a virus-membrane complex.   It is very
common to find biological activity (of enzymes for example)
associated with membrane structures and many techniques are
available for breaking up the membranes to release activity.
A typical method consists of solubilising the membrane complex
by one of many types of detergent.   However, in all instances,
the application of such techniques to the particles associated
with scrapie infectivity has not only failed to release free
virions, but resulted in a loss of infectivity proportional
to the amount of material solubilised.   This is not to say
that the particle size can never be reduced without loss of
infectivity for it has been shown with certain enzymes that
conditions may have to be defined very critically to achieve
success.   Very recently, in fact, some success has been
achieved by the use of lysolecithin as a membrane-solubilising
agent, and up to an 100-fold enrichment of scrapie infectivity
has been claimed (64).   This still however leaves an enormous
preponderance of host material associated even with the best
scrapie preparations.   So far therefore the scrapie agent
has proved sufficiently intractable to suggest that a host
membrane component is essential for infectivity.   The problem

then arises - what proportion of scrapie virion is associated
with what proportion of membrane?   Returning to the electron
microscope studies on scrapie-infected brain, the scrapie
agent would obviously be very difficult to visualize if it
consisted of a relatively small nucleic acid core or nucleocapsid strongly bonded to, or perhaps partly buried within,
tissue membrane structures.   When normal brain is homogen-
ised and filtered in the same way as scrapie-infected brain,
similar amounts of rather nondescript particles are obtained,
obviously consisting of bits of cellular structural components.   This suggests two possibilities - either the particulate suspensions from scrapie brain contain a minute population of free scrapie virions scattered amongst the host
cellular particles or the infectivity is bound to them in
some way.   The results already described suggest that the
latter alternative is more likely.

A technique commonly applied in these circumstances is
to centrifuge particulate suspensions through a succession
of solutions of different densities placed in layers on top
of each other in a centrifuge tube, or alternatively to
construct a density gradient which is continuously variable
(increasing) from top to bottom.   Sucrose solutions are
usually used up to a density of about 1.25g/ml and this may
be extended to higher densities by the addition of polysaccharides, such as Ficoll, to concentrated sucrose solutions.
When a mixture of groups of particles is centrifuged to
equilibrium on an appropriate gradient they position themselves at the place of the gradient corresponding to their
own densities.   By collection of the various layers after
this has occurred any enrichment of a particular activity
can be detected.   Such techniques applied to suspensions of

particulate material from scrapie brain have produced little or no concentration of infectivity anywhere in the gradient. A group of independent scrapie virions would have sedimented at a particular point and these results give further proof that the infectivity is in fact bound to host particulate material.

In summary the evidence seems consistent with two possibilities. Either comparatively large and irregular pieces of normal host cell membrane form an integral part of the complete scrapie virus (possibly substituting for the coat of a normal virus) or specific binding between a comparatively small viral core and host cell membrane is essential for infectivity. In the latter case the primary function of the membrane would probably be to give the right physical support rather than constitute something analogous to the viral coat. As a very rough analogy one could use the illustration of a spiders web, which depends completely on the supporting framework for its integrity and function, although the framework is an independent structure. At present there is no hard evidence favouring either of these possibilities, but we will discuss the matter further in a later section.


INACTIVATION OF THE SCRAPIE AGENT. Briefly, it now seems clear that the total destruction of scrapie activity results from treatment with powerful oxidising agents such as hypochlorite and acid permanganate solutions. Exposure to strong acids and alkalis (< pH 2 > pH 11 approximately) is equally effective. A substantial loss of titer has been found to result from exposure to iodine alcohol, 6M urea, 90% phenol, or ether. Resistance to DNAse and RNAse has

has already been mentioned.    Proteolytic enzymes have a
slight inactivating effect, but no effect has been observed
with lipase enzymes, neuraminidase of β glucuronidase.
However since the bulk of such studies have been carried out
by Hunter's group at Compton their papers should be consulted
for details (50).

In confirmation of earlier results Pattison (69) has
shown that the agent is very resistant to formalin.    For
example scrapie occurred in all of 11 goats inoculated
intracerebrally with scrapie goat brain treated for 18 hr.
at $37^o$ with concentrations of formalin ranging from 0.25-20%,
although it is not clear from these experiments how much of
the infectivity remained.

The indissoluble binding of the scrapie agent to host
cell membrane fragments introduces other complications.
Firstly it is an inevitable consequence that all scrapie
preparations subjected to inactivation procedures contain
only a minute proportion of infective agent mixed with a vast
excess of inactive material.    As Adams (2) pointed out this
may be of particular importance in attempting to assess the
heat stability of the agent.    The evidence suggests that
while inactivation of scrapie infectivity by heat begins at
about $80^o$ (or at around the melting point of DNA, as
Kimberlin and Hunter pointed out), heating to $100^o$ for
approximately 30 min results in a loss of 3-4 logs in
activity, leaving up to about 3 logs of infective residue.
This is rather exceptional stability in virus terms, but is
by no means exceptional for some types of nucleic acid.
However, it must also be borne in mind that heating a tissue
suspension in this way also results in a massive coagulation
of the protein contained in it.    Consequently the final

number of separate infective particles may depend as much
as anything on the technique of rehomogenisation.   Also, in
this, or any other inactivation procedure, it seems very
difficult to determine whether the primary effect may not
have been on the supporting membrane structures.   This will,
of course register as 'inactivation' but it may not enable
a proper comparison to be made between membrane-bound and
'free' viral agents.   Because of these problems, the dis-
agreements between different groups of workers and the
general uncertainty surrounding much of the inactivation
data relating to chemical attack on the scrapie agent, we do
not think that any purpose would be served by attempting to
make a more detailed tabulation.


IRRADIATION EXPERIMENTS.   As indicated above, the strong
association of infectivity and membrane structures increases
the difficulty of investigating the properties of the scrapie
agent.   However, there is one widely used method of estimating the approximate size of inaccessible, biologically active
sites.   This involves bombarding the material being investigated with ionising radiation under certain standard
conditions (in the dry state for example) and measuring the
associated loss in activity.   The basic theory behind this
technique is that a beam of such radiation, containing a
stream of fast moving particles, has an effect on anything
placed in its path analogous to that of a machine gun aimed
at a conventional target.   In the irradiation situation the
'target' consists of a mass of individual targets which are
the biologically active sites, and which may be dispersed
amongst a much larger quantity of inactive material.   Other
parameters remaining constant, the number of 'hits' will be

proportional to the target size, which will reflect the mass
of the active site.   If the assumption is made that a
relatively constant proportion of hits results in sufficient
damage to cause biological inactivation of individual sites,
then the size of an unknown site or molecule may be estimated
by comparison with the results obtained using biologically
active molecules of known molecular size.   However, although
this technique is simple in principle, in practice it is
fraught with difficulties and uncertainties which may
severely limit its accuracy.   Any detailed consideration of
these is beyond the scope of this volume, but they do mean
that unusual results must be looked upon with some caution.
In 1966 Alper, Haig and Clarke (11) irradiated 10mg samples
of dried scrapie brain preparations in open ampoules with a
stream of oxygen passing over them and found that unexpectedly
large radiation doses were needed to bring about any significant inactivation of the agent.   By comparison with known
standards they estimated the molecular weight of the infective
core to be no more than about $1.5 \times 10^5$ daltons.   Even if
the assumption was made that the whole of this represented
nucleic acid they rejected it as 'implausibly small' for a
nucleic acid core, and concluded that if the scrapie agent
was a virus in the conventional range its infective core
must have an extraordinary resistance to radiation.   It
must be pointed out that if target size is the principal
factor governing inactivation by this type or radiation,
then the composition of the bombarded material will be of
only secondary importance at best.   Nucleic acid, for
example, would behave similarly to anything else.   Consequently one seems forced to conclude that the only way in
which a target might be much bigger than the radiation data

indicated would be that, for some reason, an abnormally large
number of 'hits' were needed to produce inactivation.    It is
not easy to suggest how such a phenomenon might occur, unless
the target consisted of a number of infective sub-units
bound together, and if something like this did occur then
the size of the agent would essentially be that of the
individual sub-units.    However, as Adams (2) pointed out,
there seems no a priori reason why a core of the size
originally suggested by Alper et al. must be too small,
particularly if it consisted mostly of nucleic acid.    The
coding capacity would be very restricted, but as we have
seen earlier in this module, and as Adams (2) suggested
there are many possible ways by which economy might be
achieved, particularly in maximum use were made of pre-
existing host synthetic systems.    In any event the
minimum 'acceptable' size for virus cores is decreasing year
by year and recently Diener (28, 31) has produced evidence
that an infectious agent of potatoes (potato spindle tuber
virus, PSTV) contains an even smaller (RNA) core whose
molecular weight he estimates to be approximately $8 \times 10^4$
daltons (32, 75).    The most reasonable interpretation then,
of the apparent stability of the scrapie agent to ionising
radiation would seem to be that its infective core is unusually
(but not unacceptably) small but that the data give no evidence about its nature.    Since there are only three types of
biologically active macromolecules which exist in this size
range - nucleic acids, polysaccharides, and proteins, there
seems no alternative to the conclusion that the infective
core of the scrapie agent must be one of them.    Also, it is
inescapable that if there are problems over the carriage of
sufficient coding information for self-multiplication by a

nucleic acid of this size then the problems would be much greater if the core were composed of polysaccharide or protein.

A further technique is available in a situation like this, which in principle can distinguish between nucleic acids, proteins and polysaccharides in biological material. This makes use of the fact that such macromolecules vary very greatly in their ability to absorb ultra violet (UV) radiation and also in the wavelength at which maximum absorption takes place.   Nucleic acids of all types absorb UV very strongly with a peak of absorption at a wavelength of about 257nm. Proteins absorb much less strongly and the absorption peak moves to around 280nm.   Polysaccharides on the other hand absorb UV very poorly with no defined peak in this wavelength region.   Now it is obviously not possible to use this information directly to determine the composition of a minute quantity of infective agent in the presence of large amounts of cellular macromolecules of all types.   However, irradiation of macromolecules by UV results in inactivation due to the absorption of quanta of energy.   This raises the macromolecules to an excited state and, if sufficient energy is absorbed, random disintegration will result.   Among other causes, because nucleic acids absorb UV much more readily than proteins they are much more sensitive to UV induced disintegration, while polysaccharides are extremely resistant. Further, the fact already mentioned that nucleic acids and proteins absorb UV maximally at different wavelengths can be used to differentiate between them, since the inactivation observed parallels the absorption.

Consequently, it was of obvious interest to see how the scrapie agent behaved towards UV radiation and Alper, Cramp,

Haig and Clarke tried this in 1967 (10).    Using a wavelength
(250nm) fairly close to the nucleic acid absorption maximum
they showed that the scrapie agent was extremely resistant
and in fact was inactivated only to the same extent as protein
molecules with a molecular weight of around $2 \times 10^5$ daltons.
As a first approximation this result indicated that the
infective core of the scrapie agent was less sensitive by a
large factor (probably 10-100 times) than it should be if it
were composed of nucleic acid.    The conclusion was reached
that the scrapie agent was probably a self multiplying entity
not based on a nucleic acid core.

The fact that nucleic acids have a peak absorption (and
therefore of energy absorption) at 250-260nm may also be
utilised in this type of study.    In round figures about
twice as much UV radiation at this peak wavelength is
absorbed by nucleic acid than on either side, at say 240 or
280nm.    Consequently when nucleic acids, and indeed most
viruses, are irradiated with UV radiation at 240, 250-260n
and 280nm the inactivation is less at the higher or lower
wavelengths.    Latarjet, Muel, Haig, Clarke and Alper (58)
applied this principle to the scrapie agent, and an abstract
of their inactivation results in comparison with those
previously found for other viruses is shown in Table 3.    At
first sight the results obtained with the scrapie agent
appear very different from those with other viruses, but we
shall return to the problem of their interpretation shortly.
For the present, however, we will record the final, somewhat
cautious, conclusion of the authors that 'the chromophore
responsible for the UV inactivation of the scrapie agent
could be other than a part of a nucleic acid molecule or of
a nucleoprotein complex'.

Table 3

The effectiveness of the inactivation (I) of viral
agents by UV radiation of different wavelengths
(taking $I_{250}$ as 1) (after Latarjet et al.) (58).

| | Wavelength (nm) | | |
| --- | --- | --- | --- |
| | 237 | 250 | 280 |
| Various DNA and RNA viruses | 0.4-0.7 | 1 | 0.5-0.8 |
| (Average) | 0.55 | 1 | 0.65 |
| Tobacco mosaic virus $U_1$ strain | 2.3 | 1 | 0.39 |
| Scrapie agent | 6 | 1 | 1 |

Taken at their face value these results lead to two
alternatives.  Either the interpretation placed on them by
the authors is correct, in which case the scrapie agent
stands outside the framework of the currently accepted
concepts of molecular biology, or if the scrapie agent does
contain a nucleic acid core it must be shielded or protected
in some way.  A third possibility, that it may contain
nucleic acid of an unusual type which is sufficiently
radiation resistant, seems unlikely.  There is some
variation in the ability of nucleic acids to withstand UV
irradiation and, so far as DNA is concerned, factors of
single-strandedness, low thymine content, and unstacked (open)
configuration would confer a limited degree of resistance.
However it seems reasonably safe to say that at present there
is no known or theoretical structure which of itself would be
sufficiently stable.

Returning to the first alternative we must ask 'Is the scrapie agent to be the rock on which the central dogma of molecular biology must founder?'   It is obviously important not to close one's mind to the possibility that any scientific theory, no matter how well supported and entrenched, may be overturned by a single exception which it cannot accommodate.   What is at stake in this case is the proposition that only nucleic acid, and principally DNA at that, carries the coding information by which the activity of cells is governed and has the ability to specify and direct the synthesis of other macromolecules, either directly by acting as a template, or indirectly via the same process.   Thus, according to the dogma, the reverse process - by which protein or polysaccharide for example would act as a template either for the formation of nucleic acid, or for self-replication - cannot take place.

However, before concluding that the scrapie agent is an exception, as the groups involved in the irradiation experiments have (cautiously) done, let us examine the evidence from the point of view of the second alternative - that the agent does contain nucleic acid but this is protected in some way.

The point has already been made that, provided the molecular weight of that part of the scrapie agent which carries the infectivity is as small as $1-2 \times 10^5$ daltons the ionising radiation data do not conflict with the view that the core consists of nucleic acid.   So far as the UV data is concerned, although the action of this type of radiation is complex, basically it involved the absorption of energy quanta by the irradiated molecules.   Thus, when subjected to UV radiation of the appropriate wavelength, a macromolecule M changes to an excited state M* as follows:

$$M + hv \text{ (energy quanta)} \rightarrow M*$$

If the amount absorbed exceeds a certain threshold, the
vibrational energy will break the internal bonding of M and
it will fragment or disintegrate with the emission of heat
or light.  Obviously if M were originally a biologically
active molecule this process - even perhaps when only
partially completed - would inactivate it.  However, if as
is normally the case, a biologically active molecule M is
linked to other macromolecules whose integrity is not
necessary for its activity, a second possibility occurs.
The activated molecule M may protect its own structure by
syphoning off the absorbed energy ( )* to a second molecule
$M_1$ while it returns to its ground state 'M', i.e.

$$M* + M_1 \rightarrow M + M_1^*$$

This process which seems to be increasingly recognised as a
factor in the effect of radiation in biological systems, has
been termed 'intramolecular radiationless energy dissipation'.
In a classical virus the material closest to the nucleic acid
core is the protein coat (capsid).  Although little is known
of the nature of the attachment between core and capsid, the
bonding forces are weak (of the hydrogen or Van der Waals
type) and this would be likely to limit the rate at which
energy absorbed by the core could be transmitted and dissi-
pated as the bonds linking core and capsid would probably
disrupt first.  Nevertheless there are occasions when
classical viruses appear to show this phenomenon of coat
protection.  For example the $U_1$ strain of tobacco mosaic
virus (TMV) has a greater resistance to UV irradiation than
the $U_2$ strain, although the sensitivity of the free RNA
isolated from each is similar.  This is illustrated in

Table 3 where the $U_1$ strain has a pattern of sensitivity to
the three wavelengths which obviously differs from that of
DNA and RNA viruses in general.    The pattern of the $U_2$ strain
of TMV fits in with the latter group.


THEORIES ON THE NATURE OF THE SCRAPIE AGENT


On general grounds Adams and Caspary (6) suggested that
there seemed no a priori reason why the coat of a virus
should invariably consist of protein, and that a virus
composed of a nucleic acid core with a capsid consisting
largely of polysaccharide, might be stabilised to a greater
extent against inactivation by UV radiation.    Not only are
polysaccharides themselves  radiation resistant, but they
are capable of attaching to nucleic acid by the much stronger
covalent or glycosidic bonds, which should have a far greater
resiliance and ability to act as 'shock absorbers'.    Adding
this to what has already been said, the active infective
agent would consist of a nucleic acid core (approx. $10^5$
daltons) with a predominantly polysaccharide capsid (say up
to $5 \times 10^5$ daltons) specifically bonded to host membrane.
The presence of hydroxymethylcytosine instead of cytosine in
the DNA of T-even bacteriophages, and their ability to induce
hydroxymethylase enzymes in the host cell after infection,
has already been mentioned.    It is also known that the
hydroxy-methylcytosine residues in the phage DNA are linked
to glucose by covalent or glycosidic bonds.    However, the
number of glucose residues capable of sequential attachment
at each site seems to be limited to a very small number.
Consequently, although this system establishes in principle

the existence of nucleic acid-sugar residue complexes in
infectious agents, the extent to which it occurs in phage
DNA does not seem sufficient to form the basis of the
nucleic acid-polysaccharide complex proposed by Adams and
Caspary as a basis for the scrapie agent.   Further, an
attempt made to see whether scrapie infection induced the
formation of a hydroxymethylase enzyme in mouse brain was
unsuccessful (Adams, unpublished), although this may not be
entirely conclusive because the analytical techniques
available for the estimation of these enzymes were not
readily adaptable to the detection of small levels of
activity, and very little enzyme might be present in scrapie
brain.    There are, no doubt, other possibilities and recently
the nucleic acid from another phage has been shown by Marmur
and co-workers (62) to contain a large proportion of the
modified pyrimidine base 5-(4',5'-dihydroxypentyl) uracil.
This base is also able to link covalently to pentose or
glucose residues, possibly without the restrictions on the
length of the resulting side chain which seem to exist in
the case of hydroxy-methylcytosine.   Thus, although there
is as yet no direct support for the 'sugar-coated virus'
theory of Adams and Caspary, the evidence that such a concept
is a practical possibility seems to be growing.   Even though
the present systems are not entirely analogous to the Adams-
Caspary model, experiments on the radiation sensitivity of
phage-sugar residue complexes might given an indication
whether the suggestion is on the right lines.   Indeed even
the data in Table 3 may throw a little light on this.

     Although at first sight there is no clear similarity
between the results obtained with the resistant $U_1$ strain of
TMV and those with the scrapie agent, if the data are

Table 4

The effectiveness of the inactivation (I) of viral agents by UV radiation of different wavelengths (as Table 3 but taking $I_{237}$ as 1).

| | Wavelength (nm) | | |
|---|---|---|---|
| | 237 | 250 | 280 |
| Various DNA and RNA viruses (Average) | 1 | 1.82 | 1.18 |
| Tobacco mosaic virus $U_1$ strain | 1 | 0.44 | 0.17 |
| Scrapie agent | 1 | 0.17 | 0.17 |

retabulated taking the inactivation at 237nm as unity instead of at 250nm they appear as in Table 4.   This rearrangement shows a clear similarity between scrapie and the $U_1$ strain of TMV.   If in fact, the difference between $U_1$ and the other strains is due (as it seems to be) to coat/capsid protection, the scrapie results showing an even smaller relative sensitivity at 250nm might be interpreted in terms of an extension of this process consistent with a more efficient protection.

In 1968, Adams and Field (9) suggested a second mechanism by which the complete scrapie agent might have a nucleic acid core - the linkage substance hypothesis - in which incidentally the core might not have to be quite so small.   This proposal extended the 'protection' idea by removing the radiation stability of the nucleic acid core from the heart of the problem.   In essence it introduced the concept that 'infection' based on a nucleic acid containing agent could occur without the necessity of transferring

the complete infective particle from host to recipient.
This was based on two main lines of evidence.   Firstly the
well established fact that scrapie infectivity is bound to
cell membrane so tightly that all attempts to dissociate it
while retaining infectivity have failed.   Secondly, studies
by Adams, Caspary and Field indicated that there appeared to
be traces of a small DNA containing entity in the cell sap
(non-particulate) fraction of scrapie brain.   Although this
also seemed to be present in normal brain there was two or
three times as much in scrapie brain.   This particle, which
was so small that it remained in the cell sap fraction after
the application of centrifugation procedures normally
sufficient to sediment particulates, could be sedimented by
centrifugation at very high 'g' forces for prolonged periods.
Although it could not be complete scrapie agent, because of
the virtual non-infectivity of cell sap fractions prepared
in the standard way from scrapie brain, the possibility
remained that it might be a component.   Based on these
results the linkage substance hypothesis proposed the
following three component system for the development of
scrapie (shown diagrammatically in Fig. 2).

1)    A small DNA containing particle (called sub-virus
      for want of a better description), which appeared
      to contain polysaccharide also, with a probable
      total molecular weight in the region of $5 \times 10^5$
      daltons and present in the cell sap of animals
      susceptible to scrapie.   It was further postulated
      that the 'sub-virus' was capable of self-replication
      but not of causing the disease.

2)    Host cell membrane to which the sub-virus normally
      cannot bind.

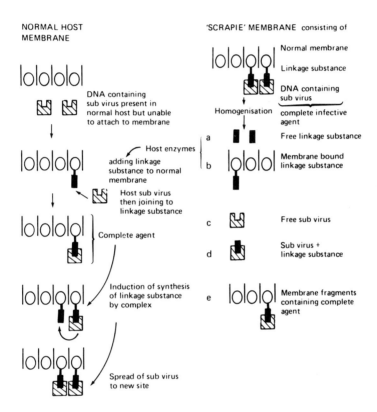

NORMAL HOST MEMBRANE

'SCRAPIE' MEMBRANE consisting of

Normal membrane

Linkage substance

DNA containing sub virus present in normal host but unable to attach to membrane

DNA containing sub virus

Homogenisation — complete infective agent

a — Free linkage substance

Host enzymes adding linkage substance to normal membrane

b — Membrane bound linkage substance

Host sub virus then joining to linkage substance

Complete agent

c — Free sub virus

d — Sub virus + linkage substance

Induction of synthesis of linkage substance by complex

e — Membrane fragments containing complete agent

Spread of sub virus to new site

Fig. 2
A diagrammatic representation of the linkage substance hypothesis of the infective process in scrapie. All fragments except (c) are considered infective if sub-virus is already present in the recipient animals. If not, only (d) and (e) are potentially infective. Fragments (a) and (d) are theoretically possible, but may be present in low concentration if the membrane-linkage substance bond is strong.
*(This figure is reproduced from the review by D.H.Adams by kind permission of the Editorial Board)*

3)    A linkage substance binding (1) and (2) together to
      form a complete infective particle which is then part
      of the membrane structure.

From the diagram (Fig. 2) it will be noted that the
further assumption must be made that the sub-virus-linkage
substance-membrane complex is capable of initiating the
production of fresh linkage substance.

As has been said, the essence of this proposal is that
it brings about a situation in which the stability of the
proposed nucleic acid core is largely irrelevant to the
problem.    The linkage substance would be the only obligatory
component for the transmission of the disease and the
initiation of the complete process for agent replication in
a susceptible recipient animal, i.e. one in which the sub-
virus was already present.    It could be a small protein or
polysaccharide, whose stability - to irradiation for example -
would then determine whether transmission could be successfully accomplished.    It must be clearly understood that the
theory does not suggest that the linkage substance is the
infective agent.    It is considered to be merely a specific
but relatively inert substance, which permits the nucleic
acid component in the sub-virus to form complete virions.
Subsequent events, including self-replication would then
proceed under the direction of the nucleic acid component.

Whether either of the hypotheses discussed above gives
a correct view of the composition of the agent, or correctly
explains its resistance to UV radiation, is still an open
question.    However, the results from the studies on UV
inactivation, which have been obtained since the linkage
substance theory was formulated, seem to make it less
necessary.    It is now clear that the other spongiform

encephalopathies are transmissable and that the responsible
agents have similar properties to scrapie (55).    Unless
scrapie is unique in some way - which is improbable - the
transmissability of the other diseases is a complicating
factor in the requirement for pre-existing sub-virus (the
genetic component) in the cells of the adaptive, as well as
the natural, hosts.    On the assumption that the linkage
substance does not determine the pattern of the disease
process, we must postulate at least four distinct sub-virus
components in, for example, squirrel monkeys to produce
scrapie, C-J disease, kuru, or TME.    Further, there would
seem to be a need for four different species of linkage
substance to select the appropriate sub-virus.    This is not
impossible, but it does mean that some mechanism of protecting or shielding the putative nucleic acid core within the
virion is a much simpler hypothesis.    However some elements
of the linkage substance hypothesis may be useful in the
consideration of other properties of the agent and these will
be discussed subsequently.

     If these or some other explanation based on nucleic
acid are not accepted, the problem is to find an acceptable
alternative.    So far as the suggestions that the infective
core may be protein or polysaccharide are concerned it must
be emphasised that there is no evidence that either of these
materials is able to function as an infective, self-replicating
unit.    The principal alternative proposition is the 'membrane'
hypothesis of Gibbons and Hunter (45) and Hunter, Kimberlin
and Gibbons (51).    This involved the concept of a steric
rearrangement of cell membranes - probably through their
sugar or oligosaccharide residues - in wuch a way that the
change propagates itself through the whole.    This is not

replication in the usual sense, but does suggest a way in
which many altered membrane units could be derived from one.
Thus, the overall process has the same appearance and end
result, as replication.   Such a system, which takes into
account the close association between infectivity and cell
membrane fragments so characteristic of scrapie, would
probably be relatively insensitive to UV, and would also fit
with the target size estimated from the ionising radiation
data if the structural alterations were concentrated into
small areas.

Further comments on the membrane hypothesis have been
made by Hunter's group (64) together with a summary of the
evidence that scrapie infectivity is closely associated with
membrane structures.

The discussion of the nature of the scrapie agent has
confined itself almost entirely, and in some detail, to the
problems posed by the irradiation data, because they are the
most striking and have attracted the most controversy.   Also,
the space limitations of this volume do not permit a general
comparison of the properties of the scrapie agent in relation
to those of other viruses.   However, a wider comparison was
made in a more general review of the topic by Adams (2), who
concluded "Although the properties of the scrapie agent are
unusual and do not allow it to be fitted into any classical
infective category, many are at least approached by other
viruses."

Before leaving the problem posed by the UV irradiation
data, let us consider some further relevant evidence, which
has arisen from the plant viruses being studied by Dr. T. O.
Diener.   Mention of the potato (PSTV) virus has already
been made, because of the evidence that it is a very small

(RNA) virus, with a core slightly smaller in fact than that
proposed for the scrapie agent.    Further results from
Diener's laboratory (30) have now shown that when purified
potato spindle tuber viroid (PSTV), tobacco ringspot virus
(TRSV), and its very small satellite (SAT) were exposed to
UV light of 254 nm the inactivation doses for PSTV and SAT
were 70-90 times larger than the dose for TRSV.    It was also
shown that the addition of clarified plant extracts to either
PSTV or TRSV made them both more resistant to UV than they
were when irradiated in pure solution.        Diener (29) has
commented on the similarities which exist between PSTV and
scrapie - notably long incubation period, apparent absence
of virions, resistance to heating, association with cellular
constituents and lack of antigenic properties.    He has also
rightly pointed out that there are very great differences
between plant viruses and those which attack the mammalian
CNS, as well as the environments in which they function, and
that any extrapolation of his results to brain must be done
with great caution.    Nevertheless it seems to us that the
results confirm the earlier suggestions which arose from the
difference in radiation sensitivity between the $U_1$ and $U_2$
strains of tobacco mosaic virus (Table 4) and also indicate
quite clearly that the reaction of some infective agents to
UV may be very different from that of others, or of purified
nucleic acid.    Precisely why some viruses should be resistant,
and others not, is unclear at present.    It seems obvious that
the nature of their capsid and coat and the immediate
surroundings is a factor, and possibly a large factor.
However, it will be recalled that although the aspect of
'target size' was considered in the discussion on ionising
radiation, no mention of this parameter has so far been made

in relation to UV.   This is partly because there seems to
be much general and theoretical confusion on this point, but
one would feel that the target size must also be taken into
account to some extent.   Apart from scrapie, PSTV and the
satellite of TRSV which are unusually small, there has been
evidence for some time that the infectious agent of hepatitis
is not only small, but also very resistant to UV radiation.
Consequently there are now four very diverse infective agents
which appear unusually resistant to UV radiation and the
most obvious characteristic they have in common is that their
(nucleic acid) cores are all exceptionally small.   Adams (2)
suggested that small nucleic acids may have an abnormal
resistance to UV radiation.   Although conventional views
appear to be that 'target size' is not a factor in UV
radiation inactivation it would seem most unlikely on general
grounds that this would hold for an indefinite range of
molecular weights.   Diener et al. (30) also discuss the
problem at some length, and again suggest that low molecular
weight nucleic acids are far more resistant to UV radiation
than those of high molecular weight.

To summarise, at present there are a number of hypotheses
concerning the nature of the scrapie agent - all of which are
more or less tenable, but a dearth of unequivocal evidence.
However, in our view, it really now is impossible to maintain
that the scrapie agent cannot be based on nucleic acid
because of its 'anomalous' resistance to UV radiation.   As
the evidence stands, it could even be that all the controversy
over the UV resistance of scrapie was a pure artefact, due to
a failure to recognise the extent to which nucleic acid can
be desensitised by a combination of small size and the protection afforded by closely associated molecules.   It may

well be that these two factors are not entirely independent. With a small core molecule, no part of it will be far away from other components of capsid and coat, which might be expected to promote energy dissipation.

On the positive side, a recent small pointer is the finding by Adams (3) of a very minute quantity of what appears to be an abnormal, low molecular weight, single stranded DNA in extracts derived from scrapie mouse brain particulates.    The work of course requires confirmation and extension to determine whether this is 'scrapie' DNA, although its presence does seem to constitute a prima facie case.

CHAPTER V


MECHANISM OF PRODUCTION OF CLINICAL DISEASE BY VIRUSES




So far we have dealt mostly with the effects of viruses
on individual cells, but the importance of a viral infection
is in the disease it produces and this, of course, involves
the whole animal.  The type and severity of a viral illness
is the resultant of the effects of the virus on the host cells
and the reaction of the host's defence mechanisms to the
foreign invader.

The most common mode of entry is via the membranes of
the conjunctiva, the nasopharynx and the gastro-intestinal
tracts.  In some diseases, such as influenza and the common
cold, the virus rarely penetrates further, but in all systemic
infections this initial stage is rapidly followed by a viraemia
during which the virus is carried to all organs of the body.
The major exceptions to this general rule are the various
arthropod-vectored viruses which are injected directly into
the blood stream.  As all the slow virus diseases are

systemic we shall not consider this aspect further, but
concentrate on how viruses actually cause disease.

The responses of the host are important factors in
disease production and these can be divided into local and
systemic reactions.   Most cells respond to the assault of
a foreign nucleic acid by producing a protein called interferon and, as viruses contain foreign nucleic acid, they are,
by and large, good inducers of interferon.   In tissue
cultures infected with a large dose of virus, interferon is
released into the culture fluids and when fresh cell cultures
from the same species are treated with this they are rendered
refractory to virus infection.   The same effect occurs in
the tissues of an infected animal with interferon being
released by the virus-infected cells into the interstitial
fluids.   In general, the amount produced by a tissue is
directly proportional to the amount of virus present.
However some "fast" viruses, such as the cytomagaloviruses
fail to stimulate interferon production.   There is, as yet,
no explanation for this phenomenon, but the presence of
cytomagalovirus in a tissue also inhibits the induction of
interferon by other viruses.   In the intact host interferon
acts as a local defense mechanism, and as the number of
infected cells increases so does the amount produced until
all the remaining uninfected cells become protected.   For
diseases to be produced, sufficient cells must be infected
before the protective action of interferon brings the spread
of virus to a halt.   Thus, the most successful disease-
producing viruses are those which are poor inducers of interferon or are able at least partially to overcome its effects.

The effect of interferon then is to abort the infection
by rendering the uninfected cells refractory to infection by

virus produced in other cells.   Consequently the effective
spread of virus from infected cells is a race between its
rate of replication and release, and the dissemination of
interferon produced at the same time.   In this sense interferon does not influence the replication rate of a virus
within individual host cells, but it does limit the final
titer of virus to a greater or lesser extent.

The second, and in some ways more important, defense
mechanism is the immune response.   Very briefly this involves
the production of lymphocytes sensitized to, and antibodies
which specifically bind to, the foreign viral antigens.
Both cells and antibodies circulate throughout the vascular
system and can therefore attack the virus at sites different
from areas of maximal replication.

In addition to the antigens which make up the nucleocapsid and envelope of the virus, the infected cells also
synthesise non-structural antigens (e.g. new enzymes) specific
for each virus.   Antibodies and sensitized lymphocytes are
produced against these cell-bound antigens and, as some are
present at the surface, the infected cells become liable to
attack by the immune response.   The mechanisms by which
sensitized cells and antibodies eliminate foreign antigens
are too complicated to give in detail here, but, in general,
antibodies bind to circulating viral antigens while sensitized
lymphocytes attack the virus-infected cells.   Antibodies
are the main factors in the recovery from poliomyelitis,
whereas lymphocytes appear to be more important in certain
togaviruses diseases.

We have seen how viruses infect animals and how the
defense systems of the host respond, but we have yet to
consider how actual disease is produced.   The most obvious

and simple mechanism is the direct cytopathic effect of the
virus on the infected cells.   Destruction of the anterior
horn cells by poliovirus results in a flaccid paralysis of
the limbs and trunk which characterises the most common form
of poliomyelitis.   This type of direct cellular destruction
is probably the most frequent cause of permanent injury and
is also a contributing factor in many of the acute illnesses
from which a complete recovery is made.   For example: -
many of the coxsackieviruses can invade heart muscle, producing areas of cellular destruction which give rise to the
clinical symptoms of myocarditis.   In most cases the immune
response rapidly eliminates the virus and the damaged cells
are replaced by regeneration from the neighbouring uninfected
muscle tissue.   However, much of the clinical 'distress' in
this and similar diseases is the result of edema produced by
leucocyte infiltration of the infected tissues.   This, of
course, is part of the host defenses directed towards the
elimination of the foreign invader.   Of necessity, this
type of disease is characterised by a short acute stage which
ends in death or an equally rapid recovery with, but more
usually without, permanent sequelae.   One might almost say
that the severity of the illness also depends upon a race
between the growth of the virus and the mobilisation of the
host defenses.   If sufficient cells become infected before
the virus is eliminated by the build up of interferon and/or
the immune response, clinical symptoms will be produced,
otherwise the infection will remain sub-clinical.   In so
far as the immune response leads to the elimination of virus-
infected cells which are essential to the integrity of the
host it may be a contributing factor in the severity of some
diseases, although probably, of course, the action of the

virus itself would eventually destroy these same cells.

One system where the immune response is in fact essential for the production of disease involves the arenavirus group, of which lymphocytic choriomeningitis virus (LCM) is the best known example. These viruses are not themselves cytopathic and infected cells produce large quantities of new infectious virus without any apparent alteration to their normal functions or replicative capacity. However, the arenaviruses do produce diseases, but only in immunologically competent animals. Mice are born before their immune mechanism can differentiate foreign from host antigens. When LCM virus is inoculated into new-born mice the virus readily replicates and spreads to all the tissues of the animals. The virus continues to be present in high and constant titer but has no significant effect on the development of the mouse. Sensitized lymphocytes are not produced at any stage, as the infected mouse appears not to recognize the viral antigens as foreign, although circulating antibodies do sometimes occur. However, if adult mice are given LCM the virus grows just as readily, but there is now a normal immune response which eliminates the infected cells. Because cells are not replaced in the tissues of the central nervous system (CNS) it is this elimination process which actually produced the CNS disease from which the virus takes its name.

Considering the slow virus diseases in the light of this complex situation several common factors become apparent. Slow virus infections of individual cells and whole tissues progress insidiously with only relatively small quantities of new virus released. Experimentally it has been found that classical interferon is either not induced by slow viruses or does not protect the cells against infection.

The slowness of the in vivo replication of the agents involved
reduces the maximum attainable levels of interferon and thus
this portion of the host defense system is effectively
negated.    Another factor common to all slow virus diseases
is the inability of the immune response to eliminate either
the infecting agent or the infected cells.    Further details
of these phenomena will be discussed in the sections dealing
with the individual virus diseases.

Tables 1 and 2 list the syndromes which fall within the
general definition of a slow virus disease and also those
diseases of presumed or postulated viral etiology which would
probably be classified as slow virus diseases if their
infective etiology were proven.    An infectious etiology has
been proved for all the diseases listed in Table 1, but has
only been postulated for those in Table 2.    The first four
diseases in Table 1 are known collectively as the spongiform
encephalopathies on account of their characteristic histo-
pathology.    The causative agents also appear to be very
similar and have been successfully transmitted to other
animal species.    All the viruses included in Table 1
replicate in several of the body tissues, but they produce
significant lesions only in the tissues named.

The spongiform encephalopathies are undoubtedly true
slow virus diseases as we have defined them, even though their
infective agents have not yet been fully characterised.    Of
the other four diseases in Table 1, two - progressive multifocal leucoencephalopathy (PML) and SSPE occur as the result
of the reactivation of latent, and possibly altered, common
viruses.    The resultant clinical pictures do, however, fit
the criteria for slow virus diseases.    Visna and maedi
appear to be neurotropic and pneumotropic variants,

respectively, of the same virus, which belongs to the leukovirus group.   Although almost all other known leukoviruses
produce tumours, usually of the reticulo-endothelial system,
in their host species, visna-maedi manifests itself as a slow
virus disease.   It is therefore included in this grouping
although the true tumour viruses, which formed a large part
of Sigurdsson's original list, are excluded.   We shall
discuss this whole question more fully in a later section.
Although certain characteristics of serum, or Australia
antigen associated hepatitis, fall into our definition of
"slow virus" diseases it is more likely to fall into a
"bridging" position between acute, persistent and slow
viruses.

There are several viruses omitted from the Tables which
have figured prominantly in earlier reviews of slow virus
diseases.   These include Riley virus, LCM and Aleutian
disease of mink.   In all cases the virus persists at high
levels for the lifetime of the host with the clinical
symptoms developing after many months due, at least in part,
to the damaging effect of large amounts of virus-antibody
complexes on such organs as the glomeruli of the kidneys.
We have already given our view that as the disease appears
to be the byproduct of a fast virus infection and not a direct
effect of the virus itself, these agents fit better into the
persistant group.

We shall now consider the evidence which may enable us
to determine the mechanisms by which slow viruses produce
slow virus diseases.   The medical aspects of the diseases
of man will be dealt with later in a separate section.

CHAPTER VI


PATHOGENESIS OF SCRAPIE


Although different strains of scrapie virus produce a
range of patterns of infection in experimentally inoculated
mice, the principal pathological features of scrapie-infected
mice are characteristic of all the spongiform encephalopathies.
Studies of the pathogenesis of scrapie, even in mice, are
expensive and time-consuming and we shall rely heavily on
the work of Eklund, Kennedy and Hadlow (37), which remains
the most comprehensive yet reported.  Their conclusions
have not been universally accepted, but the bulk of the
evidence from other workers suggests that they are basically
correct.

One week after subcutaneous inoculation of scrapie virus
into mice a significant proportion of the inoculated virus
could be detected in the spleen, but not in any other tissue.
No virus could be detected in any tissue two weeks after
infection.  Although these results have not yet been

unequivocally confirmed, it does appear that replication of
scrapie following peripheral inoculation first occurs in the
spleen following a genuine eclipse phase.

From about three weeks after inoculation virus titers
rise, first in the spleen, peripheral lymph nodes, thymus
and submaxillary salivary glands, and later spreading to
lung, intestine, spinal cord and brain.   The highest titers
of virus are found in the spinal cords and brains of sick
mice.   Scrapie virus can only be recovered from the blood
or urine of mice with great difficulty.   A similar course
of events follows intracerebral inoculation and this has led
to the suggestion that it may be necessary for scrapie to go
through a stage of replication in the lymphoreticular tissues
before gaining access to the CNS.   Separation of spleen
cells by buoyant density centrifugation indicates that blast
cells are the most probable sites of replication of scrapie
virus and that there are only two to six infectious units
per infected cell (59).

The importance of the lymphoreticular system in the
early stages of peripheral infection with scrapie is
emphasised by the observation that there is an increased
incubation period in splenectomised mice and in spleenless
mutant mice.   New-born mice show a reduced susceptibility
to peripherally inoculated scrapie.   This insensitive
period in new-born mice can be extended by treatment of the
animals with high doses of the steroid prednisone acetate,
which is a potent anti-inflammatory agent, although permanent
protection cannot be achieved (67).   When scrapie virus is
injected directly into the brains of susceptible mice neither
splenectomy nor treatment with prednisone has any marked
effect.   However, as natural infection with scrapie, and

the other spongiform encephalopathies, must occur by the
peripheral route, the apparent requirement for a replication
stage in the lymphoreticular tissues before the virus can
reach the brain is an important observation in the pathogenesis of the disease.

Although scrapie virus replicates in a wide range of
tissues the lesions are confined to the CNS and are only
observable when brain and sometimes spinal cord are examined
microscopically.   In late stages of the disease produced by
some scrapie strains the spleen appears small and "empty" of
cells, although no specific lesion is present.   The principal change observed in haematoxylin and eosin (HE) stained
sections of brain is a severe vacuolation of neuronal cytoplasm which leads to eventual destruction and complete
disappearance of the neurones with the production of a status
spongiosus of the grey matter although again the extent to
which this occurs differs considerably with different scrapie
strains.   The other characteristic lesion is hypertrophy of
the astroglial cells which is best visualised when the
sections are stained using Cajal's gold sublimate impreg-
nation.   The status spongiosus and astroglial hypertrophy
are characteristic not only of scrapie in mice, goats and
sheep, but also of the other spongiform encephalopathies.
There are considerable variations in the distribution of the
lesions within the CNS, not only between the different syndromes, but also between different types of the same syndrome
such as the different strains of scrapie.   Although astroglial cell hypertrophy is a characteristic of the spongiform
encephalopathies it is not confined to the group, but seems
to occur in response to any injury to the brain, including
acute viral infections.   However, in scrapie it is the

earliest observable pathological change and may therefore be
used to determine the presence of infection in experimental
animals.    Other important features of the pathology are such
negative observations as the absence of perivascular leucocyte infiltration, meningeal involvement and primary demyelination.    By both light and electron microscopy it has been
observed that there is a fairly widespread disruption of the
myelin sheaths, but this appears to be secondary to the
neuronal destruction.    Readers who wish to consider the
general pathological changes further are referred to reviews
by Field (40) and Gibbs and Gajdusek (46).

The absence of a leucocyte infiltration (or inflammatory
response) is only one of the unusual features of the immun-
ology of scrapie.    To date it has proved impossible to
demonstrate antibodies to scrapie virus, or scrapie-infected
cells, by any method, either in sheep or after transmission
to experimental animals.    The absence of leucocyte infiltration, even in advanced stages of the disease, indicates that
T lymphocytes are not fully sensitised either to the virus or
the virus-infected cells.    It is always possible that there
is an immune response in a small proportion of animals which
has not been observed or which we do not yet have the methods
to detect.    However, on the basis of our present knowledge
there are two possible explanations for the lack of a detectable immune response.    Firstly that the causative agent is
not recognised by the host as foreign and so does not induce
the formation of new antigens in the infected cells.
Secondly that virus-specific protein is produced in such
small quantities that the immune response is not triggered.
Both of these could be due to an almost entire dependence
on the host cell synthetic mechanisms for replication.    The

fact that inoculation of scrapie virus into a susceptible animal invariably results in death also indicates that the immune system does not respond at all and that the disease is the result of the direct destruction of neurons by the virus.

It should also be remembered that interferon has not been detected in scrapie-infected mice, nor has pretreatment of mice with interferon succeeded in reducing their suscept- ibility to the scrapie virus.  It does appear, however, that non-interferon mediated interference can occur within the spongiform encephalopathy group (23).

The inability to detect any specific response of the immune system does not appear to be due to a generalised depression of the immune mechanism.  Immunosuppressive techniques which severely damage the functions of both B and T lymphocytes do not affect the pathogenesis of scrapie, while it has been demonstrated that lymphocytes can become sensitised to scrapie-damaged tissue.


TISSUE CULTURE

Cells from normal adult brains do not grow readily in tissue culture, but glial cells can be cultured from the brains of adult animals showing clinical symptoms of kuru, C-J disease, TME or scrapie.  This is a general character- istic of virus-infected brain tissues and is not confined to the spongiform encephalopathies.  Cells cultured from infected brains release varying amounts of infectivity into the culture fluids and here again the spongiform encephalo- pathies follow the same pattern as other viruses.  However there is little or no increase in virus titer in such cultures

and in the case of scrapie it has been suggested that
replication of the virus occurs in step with the multiplication of the cells.   The infectious "particles" which appear
in scrapie brain culture fluid most probably consist of
relatively small infective units intimately bound to cell
membrane fragments.


CHEMOTHERAPY OF SCRAPIE


    In work in progress at the time of writing Adams has
studied the effects of intracerebral injections of $\alpha$-deoxy-
thioguanosine or $\beta$-deoxythioguanosine in combination with
azaserine as an inhibitor of de novo purine synthesis and of
arabinofuranosyl cytosine (Ara C) on the survival time of
C3H mice intracerebrally inoculated with     ME7 scrapie
agent.   Preliminary results have indicated that while mice
treated with either Ara C or $\beta$-deoxythioguanosine-AS died at
precisely the same time as untreated mice, those injected
with $\alpha$-deoxythioguanosine-AS have shown a slight but significant increase in survival time.


CROSSING THE SPECIES BARRIER


    The experimental evidence, so far, has indicated that
some type of close association with host membrane is an
essential factor for infectivity of the scrapie agent.
Consequently when an animal is inoculated with scrapie it
receives an infective complex containing cell membrane
belonging to the donor.   It has already been stated that
one of the common factors of slow virus diseases is the

absence of any effective immunological response.   However,
unless the scrapie donor is compatible with the new host, it
would seem very surprising if there were not some immune
response to at least the donor cell-membrane material
associated with the agent.   Further, it is most improbable
that the new scrapie 'virions' produced by replication would
continue to be associated with donor host membrane.   At some
stage therefore the infecting agent must change its membrane
'coat' from that derived from donor host to that derived from
new infected host.   Presumably then, and particularly if the
foreign membrane coat is under attack from the infected host
immune system, the membrane component will be sloughed off,
leaving a 'subvirus' particle of the type envisaged in the
linkage substance hypothesis.   Such a particle must re-
establish its specific association with components of its
new host membrane to regain its replicative capacity.   It
seems reasonable to suggest that the 'species barrier'
phenomenon (the passage from sheep to mouse for example
taking much longer than from mouse to mouse) could arise
partly because the subvirus needs time to adapt to a new host
membrane system.   Possibly the different strains of scrapie
agent which have been reported may arise because they contain
immunologically different membrane components.


RELATIONSHIP BETWEEN SCRAPIE AGENT REPLICATION AND BRAIN DNA
SYNTHESIS IN THE HOST ANIMAL

A further point to be discussed concerns the relationship between the scrapie agent and the brain tissue in which
it replicates.   Studies with classical viruses have indicated
that in at least some cases, host DNA synthesis must occur

before viral DNA begins to replicate.   Although at present
there is no information to show whether this is a necessary
prelude to slow virus replication, some studies have been
made of the incorporation of radioactively labelled thymidine
into mouse brain DNA at intervals after inoculation with the
scrapie agent.   The results have shown that this precursor
incorporates about three times as extensively into double
stranded nuclear DNA derived from scrapie brain, as into
that from normal brain.   Since only very small amounts of
precursor incorporate into normal brain DNA, this threefold
increase means little in terms of any overall increase in
brain metabolic activity.   However the change does occur at
about the time when the titer of scrapie agent begins to rise,
and morphological changes are first seen, in some brain cells.
At this point it must be made clear:-

1)    That the increased precursor incorporation into DNA is
      not associated with the replication of the scrapie agent
      itself.

2)    That it is not known whether the change is spread
      throughout the brain as a whole, or whether it is
      restricted to any particular sites, or types of
      cells, or even it if occurs only in those cells
      which have actually been infected with scrapie agent.

3)    That the change is found only in nuclear double-stranded
      DNA, there being no difference in the extent of pre-
      cursor incorporation into mitochondrial DNA between
      normal and scrapie brain.

4)    That the extent of the change in precursor incorporation
      remains relatively constant throughout the scrapie
      disease process, from its beginning about twelve weeks
      after infection, until the death of the animal.

It is very difficult to interpret these results, either in terms of the replication of the scrapie agent, or of the resulting disease process, and it is not even clear whether it has any significance at all.    It is possible that the incorporation is into the DNA of astroglial cells, which hypertrophy during the development of scrapie.    However, we have seen that this astroglial hypertrophy is a non-specific response and, since the basic data for comparison regarding precursor incorporation into brain DNA in other diseases are lacking, it is not possible to draw any satisfactory conclusions.    Similarly the incorporation may be into those cells which show an increased growth potential in tissue culture. The relationship of these phenomena to the replication of the scrapie agent is also not clear.    One seems in fact, to be left with little more than the speculative possibility that the scrapie agent cannot replicate until it has induced some, even very slight, stimulation of DNA synthesis in its host tissue.

CHAPTER VII

THE OTHER SPONGIFORM ENCEPHALOPATHIES

TRANSMISSIBLE MINK ENCEPHALOPATHY

Transmissible mink encephalopathy (TME) is a relatively uncommon disease, first observed in ranch mink in the USA in 1947. Only adult breeder animals over one year old are affected and in this group the morbidity reaches 99 to 100%. Most mink kits are killed for their pelts when six to seven months old and never develop the disease despite being housed with, suckled by, and sharing the same diet as their infected mothers. These observations, coupled with transmission experiments, indicate that TME is difficult to transmit by contact (like scrapie), although it can be acquired by the cannibalistic ingestion of flesh from diseased mink, and that the incubation period under natural conditions is at least six months. Further, following an outbreak of TME, the virus does not establish itself as endemic in the mink

farms, despite the presence of the progeny of infected
mothers.    Therefore in outbreaks of TME in mink ranches
there is little possibility that horizontal transmission
takes place and virtually no evidence for vertical transmission either.    It was therefore suggested that mink may
not be the natural host of the virus, but that it is introduced via the raw meat and offal used as food.

Following an incubation period of six to ten months
there is a slow and insidious onset to the disease with the
mink becoming increasingly excitable and then showing locomotor disturbances.    This progresses over a few weeks to
ataxia characterised by stiff, jerky movements and occasional
convulsions interspersed with periods of somnolence.    These
advanced stages of the disease last for two to six weeks,
during which self mutilation, especially of the tail, may
occur, and invariably culminate in death.    After experimental inoculation of infected tissues the mortality is 100%
and the microscopic pathology is typical of the spongiform
encephalopathies.    In the terminal stages of TME the virus
is present in brain, spleen, liver, lungs, kidney, bladder,
muscle and even feces, although the highest titer is in brain.

Experimental transmission of the virus to uninfected
mink can be accomplished by intracerebral or intramuscular
inoculation, or by feeding the animals with infected brain
material.    The incubation period reduces to four months
following intracerebral and 5-6 months following intramuscular injection, but remains at about eight months when
the infected material is ingested.    The experimental disease
is indistinguishable both clinically and pathologically from
that occurring naturally and no sex difference in incidence
has been found in any experimental series.

TME can be transmitted to a wide range of animal species, including goats, golden hamsters, albino ferrets, skunk, raccoon, and rhesus and squirrel monkeys.   Although transmission of TME to mice has been reported, those concerned now believe that the agent producing the disease in mice was a strain of mouse-adapted scrapie, introduced as a contaminant.   Transmission of clinical TME to rhesus monkeys has been achieved following passage from an apparently symptom-free rhesus monkey 33 months after injection with TME, when pathological lesions were present in the brain.   A TME-like disease developed in squirrel monkeys following parenteral inoculation of infected mink brain.   Rather surprisingly, the incubation period of TME on initial passage to skunk and raccoon was only six months, which is the same as that found for mink to mink passage.

Intracerebral inoculation of mink with extracts of certain scrapie-infected sheep brains results in the development of a disease indistinguishable from natural TME.   Disease developed after an incubation period of 12 to 14 months in all mink inoculated with an extract of Suffolk sheep brain. However, 20 months after inoculation with an extract from Cheviot sheep brain all mink remained well.   The authors (48) suggested that TME was a form of scrapie produced in mink following ingestion of infected tissues from certain strains of sheep.   One of the most interesting observations has been that TME can be transmitted to day-old hamsters, but not to 4-week-old hamsters.   This appears to be the first report of adult animals being markedly less susceptible than their young to a spongiform encephalopathy virus.   New-born hamsters are immunologically very immature, and it is to be hoped that further investigations will be made using this

system in an effort to determine whether there is an immunological reaction causing the change in susceptibility.    So
far, no in vitro immunological response has been detected in
TME, leaving it in the same position as the other members of
the group.

TME virus has not been detected in blood or circulating
lymphocytes at a time when infectious virus was present in
large amounts in lymphoid tissues such as spleen.    It has
been suggested that the TME agent can only replicate in
young, immature lymphocytes.

As might be expected from the results already given for
scrapie, glial cells taken from TME-infected mink brains have
been found to grow much more profusely in culture than normal
glial cells.    Such cultures remained infective after at
least eight passages.    The infectivity was present in whole
cells, disrupted cells and in a cell-free filtrate of the
culture fluid.    However, electron microscopic examinations
of the cultures has failed to demonstrate the presence of
typical virus-like particles and all attempts to detect
specific antibodies have failed.    Filtration studies have
indicated that TME virus is less than 50nm in diameter, but
as we have seen from scrapie, there may be some difficulty
in making any size estimations which are meaningful, because
of the possibility that what are being measured are aggregates
of virus and cell membrane.    TME has been found to be
sensitive to hot phenol and to pronase, partially sensitive
to ether, relatively resistant to 10% formalin and resistant
to UV irradiation at 254nm.    The agent will also withstand
boiling for 15 minutes.    In summary, the basic properties
of the TME virus are much less well known than those of
scrapie although it resembles these in many respects.

## THE SPONGIFORM ENCEPHALOPATHIES OF MAN

The spongiform encephalopathies of man are usually divided into two discrete clinical entities, Creutzfeldt-Jakob (C-J) disease and kuru, on the basis of their geographical distribution.

Creutzfeldt-Jakob (C-J) disease is the name given to those cases which occur sporadically in man throughout the world and was first described in the 1920s. It has an insidious onset, followed by progressive mental deterioration and leads to death in 6 months to two years. Males and females are equally susceptible with the majority of cases occurring between 35 and 65 years of age. The clinical manifestations and the distribution of the histological lesions in the brain vary quite markedly from patient to patient, suggesting that C-J is not a single entity, but a group of closely related diseases.

The most unusual aspect of kuru is its restriction to the primitive Fore people who occupy a region in the Eastern Highlands of New Guinea. This area had little contact with Europeans before 1947 and although it is mentioned earlier, the disease was first accurately described in 1957. Kuru appears to have been prevalent in the Fore people for at least 50 years and in the 1957 description was predominantly a disease affecting children and adult women. Since then the overall incidence has almost halved and it has virtually disappeared among children under 12 years of age. During the period prior to contact with Europeans the Fore people practised ritual cannibalism of their dead relatives, during the course of which the women and children became thoroughly contaminated with the brain tissues. This practice is

believed to be extinct now and the changing pattern of
incidence appears to be directly related to the end of these
rituals.   The epidemiological data indicates a minimum
incubation period of four years extending, in a significant
number of cases, to 20 years or more.   Vertical transmission
of the disease from mother to child also appears to be a
possibility and the idea that the Fore ethnic group is a
fertile ground for the virus is gaining considerable support.
The passage of time will now tell us if the spread of the
disease was entirely due to cannibalism or if there is some
other, as yet undetected, mode of transmission.   It may be
said here that not everyone accepts the cannibalism theory,
and it has been claimed that it is possible to explain the
disease incidence in purely genetic terms.   However the
recent successful transmission of kuru to primates does
seem to establish its basically infective nature.

Since 1965 successful transmission of kuru has been
achieved from the brains of 11 patients to 18 chimpanzees,
with an incubation period varying from 14 to 39 months.   The
method of inoculation was intracerebral often in conjunction
with a peripheral route.   The disease has also been transmitted to one chimpanzee following a combination of intracerebral and multiple peripheral inoculation of pooled
visceral tissues from two other kuru patients.   The kuru
virus can be serially passaged in chimpanzees following intracerebral or peripheral inoculation of infected brain, with
the mean incubation period in the former series reducing to
11 months from the 22 months of the primary transmission.
The virus can also be detected in pooled visceral tissues
from infected chimpanzees.   Primary transmission of kuru to
several species of new-world monkeys (capuchin, woolly,

spider and squirrel) has also been accomplished with incubation periods of 20 to 50 months and to a rhesus monkey after
100 months.    Serial passage of kuru from chimpanzees and
new-world monkeys to new-world monkeys has also been shown,
but the incubation period has remained long, the only exception being passage from capuchin to capuchin monkey in 10 to
13 months.    The clinical picture in all the experimental
primates is very uniform and closely resembles the human
disease.    So far it has not proved possible to transmit the
disease to any animals other than primates.

The transmissible nature of C-J disease was demonstrated
in 1967 by the inoculation of brain material into chimpanzees
and several species of new-world monkeys.    In a series of
42 chimpanzees inoculated with brain extracts from 26 patients,
18 animals became ill.    The incubation period following
intracerebral inoculation ranged from 11 to 16 months and it
has also proved possible to transmit the disease by peripheral inoculation with an incubation period of 16 months.
Serial transmission from chimpanzee to chimpanzee has been
accomplished but with virtually no decrease in the incubation
period which is unusual in this group of agents.    Transmission from man direct to squirrel, spider and capuchin
monkeys took much longer, with incubation periods ranging
from 23 to 29 months.    Passage from chimpanzees to squirrel,
spider, capuchin or woolly monkeys occurs following incubation periods of 9 to 28 months.    The general pattern of the
illness in experimentally infected primates is similar to
that in man.    So far C-J virus has been recovered only from
brain and not from visceral tissues.

Recently, Duffy and his colleagues (34) reported the
occurrence of C-J disease in a 56-year-old woman eighteen

months after receiving a corneal transplant from a man who
was found (after the transplant had been performed) to have
been suffering from C-J disease.   The donor died of intercurrent pneumonia and C-J disease was not diagnosed until
autopsy.   Although this single case does not provide sufficient evidence to say unequivocally that C-J virus was
present in the cornea, the known rarity of the disease
suggests that this was the most probable explanation.

Virus-like particles have been observed by electron
microscopic examination of biopsy material from two patients
with C-J disease.   The particles were of two types - myxo-
virus-like and papovavirus-like, but the etiological significance is completely unknown, and indeed other extensive
examinations have failed to reveal any recognisable virions
in human or animal brains.   However, specific changes have
been observed in infected brains which are very suggestive
of the effects of viral replication.

The pathology of the brains from all the kuru-infected
primates is remarkably constant and is very similar to the
disease in man.   Electron microscopic examination of human
and chimpanzee brain has failed to reveal any virus-like
particles, but once again the changes are suggestive of the
effects of a viral infection.   Cultures of cells from kuru-
infected chimpanzee brains grow very readily and the virus
persists in such cultures for at least 70 days at 37°C.
Attempts to demonstrate the presence of interference in these
cultures (and those from C-J infected chimpanzees), using a
range of indicator viruses, were completely negative.   It
should be mentioned here that many of the chimpanzee tissue
cultures were infected with latent viruses which emerged on
prolonged in vitro growth.   There is no evidence to connect

any of these agents with the etiology of kuru.

Similarly, cells can be grown readily from C-J infected human and chimpanzee brain tissues in vitro.  Homogenates of these explant cultures have been used to transmit C-J disease to two chimpanzees following intracerebral inoculation.  In the first case the cells were grown from a chimpanzee for one month while in the second the cells were cultured for 255 days from human autopsy material.  The cultures were maintained at $37^{\circ}C$ and the incubation period was about 16 months.  It is not known whether this represents actual replication of the agent in the cultures or only persistence of pre-existing virus.

Despite the difficulties involved in working with chimpanzees, some of the basic properties of the kuru virus (and to a lesser extent C-J virus) have already been elicited. Suspensions of kuru virus, such as phosphate buffered saline homogenates of brain tissue, remain viable indefinitely at $-70^{\circ}C$, or after lyophilization, and are not appreciably reduced in disease producing ability following heating at $85^{\circ}C$ for 30 minutes.  Human kuru brain tissue contains at least $10^7$ infectious doses per gram while in infected chimpanzee brain titers greater than $10^{8.5}/g$. have been found. Both viruses pass through 220 nm APD filters but have not been detected in filtrates of smaller APD filters.  Neither virus has been detected in whole blood, serum, urine, CSF, milk, placenta or amniotic fluids of kuru or C-J patients or infected primates.  So far no chimpanzee has developed kuru following ingestion of infected brain, but this might require an extended incubation period.  Treatment of kuru-infected chimpanzees with artificial double-stranded RNA capable to inducing interferon production has had no apparent effect on the course of the disease.

No specific antibodies directed against C-J or Kuru
viruses or kuru-infected cells have been demonstrated by
neutralization, complement fixation or immunofluorescence
tests.    Attempts to precipitate kuru virus as an antigen-
antibody complex using serum from infected and "hyperimmun-
ized" primates and antigammaglobulin have also proved negative.
Similarly, no deposits of complement, gammaglobulin or virus-
antibody complexes have been detected in serum or in frozen
sections of brain, kidney or other tissues from infected
primates or kuru patients.    Sera from C-J and kuru patients
and inoculated primates have been screened for antibodies to
over 50 viruses, but no significant or meaningful pattern of
antibodies has been found.    Kuru is very similar in all
respects, except the clinical presentation, to C-J disease.
It has been postulated that kuru may have developed in the
Fore people by transmission of the virus from a sporadic case
of C-J disease to the relatives of the patient following his
ritual cannabalisation.

# CHAPTER VIII

## PROGRESSIVE MULTIFOCAL LEUKOENCEPHALOPATHY

Progressive multifocal encephalopathy (PML) is a rare disease of the CNS, characterised by proliferation of glial cells and demyelination, which usually occurs as a late clinical complication in patients with chronic lymphocytic leukemia or Hodgkins disease. Although PML has been observed in otherwise apparently normal persons, there is an underlying malignant lymphoproliferative disease in over 50% of the cases. Non-lymphoid malignancies and benign diseases of the reticulo-endothelial system form the background to the remainder of the earlier reported cases. The majority of these patients had received varying doses of X-irradiation, cytotoxic drugs, and/or adrenal corticosteroids. It is therefore of considerable significance that some recent cases of PML have occurred in patients undergoing immunosuppressive therapy.

PML is a disease of advancing age, with the majority of cases appearing during the fifth to seventh decades of life. The youngest recorded patient was 28 years old at the time of death while the oldest was 84, and males are affected more commonly than females.   In many cases the underlying disease is itself fatal and this obscures the extent to which PML contributes to the death of these patients, although in the absence of any other disease death can be wholly attributed to the PML.   The average duration of the disease in all patients is three to six months although it may sometimes extend to over twelve months.   Typical, but minimal PML lesions have been observed at autopsy in the absence of clinical symptoms during life, but it is not known whether these represent an incipient stage or an abortive form of the disease.   The principal neurological signs of PML are mental changes and motor disturbances, and at autopsy it is found that the extent and topography of the pathological lesions correlate very well with the symptomatology and duration of the illness.   The lesions are characterised by necrosis and demyelination and, despite its name, the disease is really a multifocal encephalomyelopathy and not a multi-focal leukoencephalopathy.

The outstanding cytological feature of early lesions, which appears to be specific for this disease, is the presence of large numbers of altered oligodendroglial cells.   The nuclei of these cells are enlarged and basophilic, the regular chromatin pattern is lost, and many contain inclusions which may be basophilic, eosinophilic or amphophylic.   The basophilic inclusions stain intensely for DNA.   Giant astro-glial cells are the main feature of the later, more advanced lesions.

The presence of the inclusion bodies suggested that a virus might be the etiological agent and this inevitably led to a retrospective study of the formalin-fixed material in the electron microscope.  Virions, with the general characters of the papovavirus group, were found in the distended oligodendroglial nuclei.  In early lesions they were present in up to two thirds of the glial cell nuclei, but were rarely seen in the late lesions.  Virions were occasionally found in astroglial cells, but never in neurons, endothelial cells, macrophages or giant cells.  The majority of the virions appeared round or hexagonal with a diameter of 33-38nm, but oblong particles were also seen.  Due to the poor quality of the fixation procedures it was impossible to obtain an accurate estimate of the size.  Virions were sometimes found in the cytoplasm, but always in association with intranuclear particles, while in some preparations they appeared to be associated with myelin sheaths.  Examination of partially purified preparations by negative contrast indicated a particle size of 41nm which is similar to the polyomavirus genus of the papovaviridae.  Similar investigations of control materials were all negative and by the beginning of 1971 it seemed reasonably established that papovavirions were present in all adequately studied cases of PML, mainly at the sites of initial tissue injury. Further, during 1971 and 1972 two independent groups of workers reported the isolation of cytopathic papovaviruses from the brains of three separate cases of PML.  In view of the significance of these results in the possible future elucidation of a viral etiology for the diseases listed in Table 2 we shall recount in detail the techniques used by both groups for the isolation of their agents.

   ZuRhein (83) and her colleagues (68) obtained autopsy
specimens of early brain lesions from a patient with an eight
year history of Hodgkins disease who died four months after
the onset of typical PML.   Papovavirus were seen in the
electron microscope and cultures of primary human fetal brain
(containing astroglial cells either alone or with spongioblasts)
were inoculated with extracts of the brain lesions.   Following 30 days incubation, the astroglial cells were stained and
found to contain some enlarged cells which had bizarre, deep-
staining nuclei.   No CPE or inclusions were seen, but control cultures did not contain the unusual nuclei.   The
effect could be transmitted to fresh astroglial cells by
freezing, thawing and sonicating the affected cultures but
without any change in the incubation period.   However, when
cultures containing spongioblasts (PHFG cells) were inoculated
with brain lesion or astroglial cell culture extracts, a CPE
was observed in 10 or 12 days.   The infected cultures contained mounds of normal cells together with cells in mitosis,
necrotic cells and cells with compact intranuclear inclusions.
The PHFG cells were either destroyed or altered so as to be
unrecognisable and large numbers of virions were seen in these
cultures.   The average particle size was about 42 nm when
examined by negative contrast and 39 nm when positively
stained and examined by thin sectioning.   When titrated in
PHFG cultures the titer of the virus (now referred to as
strain JC) was found to be greater than $10^6 TCD_{50}$ (50% tissue
culture infective doses)/g of brain.   PHFG cells infected
with the virus were not stained by fluorescein-conjugated
antisera to SV40, polyoma or human papilloma viruses,
although SV40 virus gave a similar CPE in PHFG cells.
   In the second communication, Weiner and his co-workers

(79) reported the isolation of papovaviruses from two cases
of PML.   The first case was a 55-year-old woman who had a
four month history of progressive, bilateral, focal neurologic
signs.   A biopsy of the right frontal lobe showed typical
histological lesions of PML, but no virions were seen in the
limited amount of material which was available for electron
microscopy.   The second case occurred in a 38-year-old
woman with systemic lupus erythematosus who had been treated
with steroids and cyclophosphamide and who died 20 months
after the onset of a progressive right sided hemiparesis.
An autopsy was performed 4 hours after death and the brain
showed typical histological lesions of PML and virions 33-35
nm in diameter.   Primary cultures of pleomorphic cells were
obtained from the brains of both cases.   The cultures were
sub-cultured every 7-10 days and a CPE was observed at the
sixth passage from the first case, the cells showing a heaped
appearance and loss of contact inhibition.   These cells were
fused with African green monkey kidney cells (GMK) but the
heterokaryons showed no CPE.   Homogenates of the heterokaryons were passaged to fresh GMK cells and at the second
pass a CPE consisting of cytoplasmic vacuolation followed by
cell lysis developed in 10 days.   The CPE could be serially
passaged, but the apparently transformed brain cell line
failed to grow after 20 passages.   In case 2 the second
sub-culture of the brain cells was fused with GMK cells and
homogenates of the heterokaryons produced a CPE in GMK cells
after 7-10 days.   Homogenates of the third sub-culture of
the brain cells gave a CPE in GMK cells directly, without
fusion, in the same time.   No CPE was observed when homogenates of the original brain tissues were inoculated into GMK
cells nor could any similar agents be recovered from cells

grown from the brains of patients without PML.   Electron
microscopy of thin sections of third passage brain cells
failed to show any virions, but sections of GMK cells infected
with the isolates showed the presence of 33-35nm diameter
particles packing the nuclei.   In negative contrast, typical
papovavirions of 42nm were seen.   GMK cells infected with
either of the two isolates showed specific nuclear fluorescence with sera from case 1, SV40 antiserum, and rabbit
antisera prepared against both isolates.   In many cells the
fluorescence included the nucleolus which is an atypical
finding for SV40 virus.   Frozen sections from the brain of
case 2 showed similar nuclear fluorescence of some cells
surrounding the white matter lesions.   Although both SV40
antiserum and serum from case 1 specifically stained the cells,
a greater proportion were stained by the human serum.   Serum
from case 2 did not stain infected cells but this was probably
due to the suppression of antibody production by the cytotoxic drugs with which the patient was being treated.   By
cross-neutralisation both the isolated and SV40 viruses
appeared identical and neither isolate agglutinated human or
guinea pig erythrocytes, which is also characteristic of SV40
virus.   An identical agent was successfully re-isolated in
PHFG cells from the brain material of case 2 and the authors
concluded that the two isolates were not contaminants from
the GMK cells.   Despite the close relationship to SV40
there was no history of previous infection with SV40 virus
in either case.

The results of these investigations indicated that the
etiological agent of PML was indeed a polyomavirus probably
related to the simian agent SV40.   Very little is known
with any certainty of the number and incidence of these

viruses in the general population and another recently
isolated human variant of SV40 virus has further confused
the situation.   This strain (BK) was recovered from the
urine of a patient into whom a kidney and ureter had been
transplanted three months previously, and who was in the
process of rejecting the transplanted ureter.   The BK virus
showed low-level serological cross-reactions with SV40 virus,
but grew much more slowly in tissue culture and agglutinated
human group O and guinea pig erythrocytes.   Low levels of
specific antibodies were present in both the donor and
recipient before the transplant, and these rose in the
recipient following the onset of rejection.   The authors
(43) believed that the virus was reactivated either in the
patient or in the transplanted kidney and ureter, probably
as a result of the concomitant immunosuppressive therapy.
They also suggested that necrosis in the transplanted ureter,
secondary to rejection, might have provided a suitable site
for the initial virus replication.   However, as virus
continued to be excreted in the urine for at least a month
after removal of the donor ureter, there must have been
another site of replication which was not identified.

Other workers have now recovered polyomaviruses in
human fetal glial cell cultures from cases of PML in different parts of the world.   Studies on these strains of human
polyomavirus, SV40 virus and mouse polyoma virus itself,
using immunofluorescence and electron microscopical
agglutination tests, have shown the existence of at least
three distinct antigenic sub-types of SV40 virus.   All the
human strains are quite distinct from mouse polyoma virus,
but cross-react to a greater or lesser extent with SV40
virus when sera from hyperimmunised rabbits are used.   If

early rabbit antisera are used, Weiner's two original strains
are indistinguishable from SV40 virus whereas the JC and BK
strains are distinct from each other and SV40 virus.    The
majority of PML cases so far studied are associated with JC
virus, only two with SV40 virus and so far none with BK virus.
The human strains of SV40 virus show minor differences in
nucleic acid content when compared with the classical
laboratory strain.

Antibodies to JC virus are present in about 70% of
adults, while BK virus is at least as prevalent, with 50% of
children of three years of age having antibody.    Antibodies
to SV40 virus are present in only small numbers of the
"normal" population, but in over 20% of people who received
polio vaccine before the presence of SV40 virus as a contaminant was known.    There were no major clinical differences
between the PML cases associated with SV40 and JC viruses.
All three antigenic types produce tumours in hamsters.    No
demyelinating lesions have been found but JC virus appears to
be the first virus more oncogenic in brain than in extra-
neural tissues.

A consistent feature of all cases of PML is a deficiency
in cell-mediated immunity, although production of antibodies
may be normal.    In vitro SV40 is a relatively slow growing
virus and the PML strains are even slower than usual.    The
suggestion has been made that the "slow" step in SV40 synthesis could be a requirement for the presence of functional
capsid protein for maturation of the double-stranded DNA,
although this suggestion must be considered in the light of
the discussion in the earlier chapters.    It therefore
appears probable that PML results from the slow replication
of a human polyomavirus following the activation of a latent

infection brought about by the crippling of the immune response.   The multifocal nature of the lesions is very suggestive of infection of the CNS following a viremia and it is
therefore possible, if not probable, that the latent infection is not of the CNS, but of an as yet unidentified site
where the activation and initial replication occurs.

At least four patients have been treated with antiviral
drugs known to be active against DNA viruses.   One patient
treated with idoxuridine and two treated with cytarabine
(Ara C) died, although there was an immediate but short-
lived period of remission in one of the latter.   However,
the fourth patient, who had been treated for the previous
four years for chronic lymphocytic leukemia, made an almost
complete recovery following a course of cytarabine therapy
and remained well at his last attendance ten months after
treatment.   It therefore appears that under the right circumstances PML can be successfully treated with antiviral agents.

# CHAPTER IX


## VISNA-MAEDI


Visna and maedi are neurotropic and pneumotropic types of the same virus, the names being derived from the CNS and lung diseases in Icelandic sheep with which they were originally found to be associated.  Indeed, visna has only been found in Iceland and Holland, but diseases similar to maedi have been found in many parts of the world.  The first description of the pneumotropic disease was given by Marsh in 1923 (63) relating to a progressive pneumonia of Montana sheep.  However the first successful isolation and characterisation of the causative virus of maedi was achieved by the Icelandic group (72) and this name has now been accepted for the pneumotropic variant.  Visna disease was not recognised until some time later, but as most laboratory studies have been carried out on this variant of the virus we shall follow Andrewes and Pereira (12) and give visna priority.

In nature, visna has an insidious onset and never occurs
in sheep under two years of age,  The first sign is stumbling,
associated with weakness of the hind limbs.  The animals tend
to lose condition, and trembling of the lips and eyelids may
be seen.  There is a gradual deterioration of the ability
to use the limbs, which causes difficulty in walking, and may
end in complete paralysis.  The animals remain afebrile
throughout and the course of the disease is always protracted,
sometimes with periods of partial remission.  The duration
from the onset of symptoms to the inevitable death ranges
from a few months to several years, giving rise to the name
'visna' which means 'wasting'.  At autopsy no specific
macroscopic lesions are found while the microscopic changes
are best described as a meningo-leukoencephalitis.  The
initial lesion is a meningeal or subependymal infiltration
and proliferation of cells of the reticulo-endothelial
system.  In advanced cases, foci of microglial infiltration
are found throughout the white matter of the brain and brain-
stem.  The larger lesions tend to necrose and form cavities
with moderate demyelination as a frequent secondary change.
Extensive perivascular cuffs of lymphocytes, plasma cells
and histocytes are found in the vicinity of the lesions.
Following intracerebral inoculation of healthy sheep with
infected brain material there is a latent period of one to
two months when no virus can be detected.  This is followed
by a sub-clinical stage of about six months duration, when
there is a marked increase in the number of white cells in
the CSF, and visna virus can be recovered from CSF, whole
blood (chiefly from leukocytes) and saliva.  In some animals
the cell count returns to normal after several months and
these animals never show clinical symptoms.  In other cases

the cell count remains high and signs of paralysis appear.
Once clinical signs are seen the disease progresses relent-
lessly to death.    Virus can be recovered from many organs in
addition to brain, both at death, and several months earlier
during the sub-clinical stage when typical brain lesions are
often present.    Complement fixing antibodies are formed a
few weeks after infection, and neutralising antibodies after
some months.    The role played by antibodies in the course
of the disease, if any, is unknown, but it does appear that,
as with the other slow virus diseases the immune response to
visna virus is deficient (73).

Maedi and similar pneumonic diseases occur much more
frequently than visna, although the epidemiologies of both
are closely related.    The first clinical signs of maedi are
listlessness and loss of condition, which often becomes
apparent when the weather changes for the worse, or after the
sheep have been exposed to any unusual physical stress.
Another early sign is laboured and difficult breathing,
while after exertion the respiration becomes very rapid and
shallow.    The temperature remains normal, despite the
raised respiration rate.    As the disease progresses the
breathing becomes more laboured and the blood haemoglobin
level decreases.    In nature the disease is only found in
animals more than three to four years old and the duration
is usually between three and six months, although some
animals survive for up to a year.    As it is usually the
policy to slaughter infected animals, it is difficult to
make a precise estimate of the average duration.    In
animals which are allowed to survive, death is usually due
to a secondary bacterial pneumonia.    At autopsy, macroscopic
changes are only found within the chest cavity, the lungs

being grossly enlarged with diffusely thickened tissues.
The increase in size is much less marked than the increase
in weight which may be two to four times that of normal lungs.
The lymph nodes associated with the lungs are always enlarged,
while characteristically, lymphoid follicles are present on
the surface of the lung.    In some respects the disease
resembles a lymphoma.    Microscopically the main lesion is a
chronic interstitial inflammation with thickening of the inter-
alveolar walls due mainly to monocytic and lymphocytic infiltration.    In advanced cases, complete obliteration of the
alveoli may occur.    Hyperplasia of the smooth muscle in the
interalveola walls and the epithelium in the smooth bronch-
ioles is also found.    In giemsa-stained smears from maedi-
infected lungs there are almost always large mononuclear cells
containing characteristic inclusion bodies.    Maedi can be
transmitted to healthy sheep by intrapulmonary, intranasal,
or intravenous inoculation of the virus and apparently also
by feeding and contact.    The incubation period is about two
years although lung lesions are detectable as early as one
month after infection.    A leukocytosis is also present for
about one year prior to the onset of symptoms and virus can
be isolated from the leukocytes, CSF and various organs.
The antibody response is similar to that of visna, and
antigenically the two viruses are closely related if not
identical.    In fact, intrapulmonary inoculation of maedi
virus sometimes produces not only typical maedi but also a
neurological disease indistinguishable from visna.    This
supports the view, first suggested by the epidemiology, that
visna is a neurological variant of maedi.

    Epidemiological observations of the naturally occurring
progressive pneumonias indicate that although maedi is a

contagious disease, its communicability is very low while the
sheep are on pasture, but is greatly enhanced by close contact
during winter housing.   Transmission can occur by contamination of the drinking water with feces from infected animals.
During the sub-clinical period the disease is rarely transmitted except from mother to lamb.   Once the disease is
introduced into a flock of sheep it becomes endemic with a
mortality rate of 20-30% per annum.   Although a certain
degree of genetically determined susceptibility occurs, the
only accepted method of eradication so far is a policy of
slaughtering all sheep in an infected area.

The first cases of visna in Iceland were seen in sheep
which also showed the symptoms of maedi in varying degrees
of severity.   The incidence of visna in these flocks increased
until in some areas the mortality due to the visna variant
was greater than that due to maedi.   Visna did not arise in
all maedi-infected flocks, but only in those in which maedi
had been endemic for long periods.   Outside Iceland,
although maedi-like diseases are widespread, it is only in
Holland that occasional cases of a visna-like meningo-
encephalitis have been found in flocks affected with
Zwoegerziekte (the Dutch name for their progressive pneumonia).   All of the evidence therefore supports the view that
visna is a late variant of maedi.

The causative viruses have been recovered from visna,
maedi, zwoegerziekte, progressive pneumonia in Montana and
from affected sheep in West Germany and Denmark.   All
strains are related antigenically, with the pneumotropic
isolates showing greater diversity than those from cases of
visna.   In experimental cases of visna-maedi running a
protracted course the antigenic characters of the virus

appear to alter in the continued presence of the host defences.
However, for all practical purposes the strains as a whole can
be considered to be minor variants of the same virus.    A
serological relationship has also been found between visna-
maedi and progressive pneumonias of sheep in many other parts
of the world, even though the causative virus has not yet
been recovered.   In vitro, growth of visna-maedi occurs in
cells derived from pigs and cattle in addition to sheep, but
most work has been done using cultures of sheep choroid
plexus cells.   Following infection of these with tissue
culture-adapted virus there is a latent period of about 16
hours, followed by a rapid increase in the production of new
virus over a further 16 hours or so.   After about another
four days, during which some new virus is produced, the cell
sheet undergoes extensive degeneration.   The initial cytopathic effect is syncytia formation followed by cellular
degeneration which is similar to that brought about by measles
virus.   The production of syncytia is a direct effect of the
virions on the cells and does not require active viral
replication.   Immunofluorescent studies have shown that
visna virus antigens are formed in the cytoplasm and then
accumulate at the cell surface, and electron microscopy has
shown that new virions are formed by budding from the cell
surface.   These are spherical particles with an average
diameter of 85nm and appear very similar to those of certain
RNA tumor viruses or leukoviruses.   All strains are equally
sensitive to chloroform, ether, metaperiodate, trypsin,
formaldehyde (0.04%), UV radiation and heating to $56^{o}C$.
However, maedi virus was inactivated three times more rapidly
at pH 4.2 than was visna virus.   Replication of visna-maedi
virus is inhibited by the presence of 5-bromodeoxyuridine and

and by actinomycin-D while the virion contains a reverse
transcriptase enzyme system.   This indicates that although
the visna-maedi virion contains single-stranded RNA, replication can only occur by an initial reverse transcription of
this RNA to double-stranded DNA and not by direct RNA replication.   These properties place visna-maedi within the
leukovirus group and we shall now examine the similarities
in detail.

No antigenic relationship has been demonstrated between
visna-maedi and any leukovirus.   However, the protein pattern
obtained by polyacrylamide gel electrophoresis of purified
visna virus shows some similarity to that found in members
of the leukovirus group.   Analysis of the nucleic acid
component of purified visna virions has shown the presence of
two components - a major one of 63s single-stranded RNA, and
a smaller one of 4-7s.   This is very similar to the composition of the nucleic acid of other leukoviruses, but the
visna 63s component is more heterogeneous than that of the
tumor group.   A further difference is that in the other
leukoviruses the small RNA component is believed to be derived
from host-cell material, whereas in visna it appears to be
virus specific.

The final proof, if such were required, that visna-maedi
was a genuine member of the leukovirus group came when it was
shown that at least two strains were able to transform murine
cells in vitro and that these cells were then able to produce
tumors in vivo.   Despite this however, there is no evidence
that visna-maedi is the cause of any tumors in sheep.

It may then be asked why visna-maedi infection results
in the development of slow virus diseases but not tumors?
In the first place, if the pathology of the progressive

pneumonias is closely studied, it is obvious that they share
many features with virus-induced tumors.  The pathogenicity
of the virus appears to be due to the replacement of the air-
spaces in the lungs by cellular infiltration or hyperplasia.
The similarity to a virus-induced tumor is increased by the
absence of any degenerative lesions, although the monocytes
at least, contain viral inclusions which are typical of a
lytic infection and are not seen in transforming infections.
It therefore seems that maedi occupies a position between the
'lytic' type of disease where cellular destruction is produced as a direct consequence of the virus infection, and a
true tumor.   Visna, on the other hand, has much more the
appearance of a typical slow virus disease, resembling SSPE
in many ways, with the primary lesion producing a necrotic
change.   We may then summarise the situation by saying that
while visna belongs in the slow virus group, maedi occupies
a 'bridging' position between the slow virus diseases and
the virus induced tumors.   Why such different diseases are
produced by apparently similar viruses is an important
question for future investigations.


TUMOR VIRUSES


    At this stage it is probably advisable to say a few
words about the tumor viruses and to explain why, despite
their inclusion by Sigurdsson in his original classification,
we consider them to belong to a group quite separate from
the slow viruses.   Some of these differences were touched
on in relation to visna-maedi.   However to enlarge briefly
upon what was said, when tumor viruses infect suitable host
cells they do not only produce a cytopathic effect, but

transform (a proportion of) the non-lysed cells into tumor
cells.    These transformed cells contain a combination of the
genomes of both virus and host.    In the case of the DNA-
containing viruses, like the papovaviruses, the viral DNA is
incorporated directly into the host-cell genome, while in the
case of leukoviruses the RNA is first transcribed into DNA.
The reverse transcriptase enzyme system produces first an
RNA-DNA hybrid from the viral RNA and then a second enzyme
transforms the hybrid into double stranded DNA.    This DNA
provirus can then act either as the template for the production of viral RNA or become integrated into the host cell
genome.    The transformed cells are capable of continuous
growth both in vivo and in vitro.    In vivo, they give rise
to tumors from which the animal ultimately dies - unless
eliminated by the host's immune mechanism.    The replication
of the virus is not necessary for this unrestrained growth.
Indeed, in well established tumors, infectious virus cannot
be detected by direct methods, although it can often be
induced by fusing the tumor cells with highly permissive
indicator cells.    It is therefore clear that the disease in
the animal is not, as has already been said a direct consequence of virus-induced cell destruction.    The death of the
animal occurs as a result of the invasion of the tissues by
the new entity:- the hybrid  virus-host-cell, and its
relentless progression as such, the hallmark of the disease
known as cancer.    The term 'relentless progression' or
'inexorable process' has already been applied to describe
the events in a slow virus disease, and perhaps emphasises
the similarity in the general effect on the host of both
slow and tumor viruses.    However it should be clear by now
that slow viruses produce progressive, degenerative lesions

which appear to be due to a direct effect on the host cells
and, as was included in our definition, that the severity
of the disease is related to the increase in virus produced.
These are the essential reasons why tumor viruses must be
placed in a separate category.

For those interested, reference may be made to reviews
by Eckhart (35) and by Temin (77).

CHAPTER X

SUBACUTE SCLEROSING PANENCEPHALITIS

Subacute sclerosing panencephalitis (SSPE), or Dawson's inclusion body encephalitis, is a disease of children and young adolescents with an estimated incidence of about one in a million.   It is characterised by an insidious onset of behavioural changes and decline of intellectual ability. The illness usually lasts from three months to two years, but sometimes runs a more protracted course of up to six years.   Although the patients remain afebrile, the pathology of the early lesions is characteristic of a viral encephalitis. As the disease progresses the general histopathological pic- ture becomes one of diffuse perivascular inflammation, neuronal degeneration, glial cell proliferation and a variable degree of demyelination.   As the name given to the disease by Dawson indicates, the chief cytological feature is the presence of eosinophilic intranuclear and cytoplasmic inclusion bodies.   The nuclear inclusions are typical

Cowdry type A with the result that herpes simplex virus was first postulated as the etiological agent. However, electron microscopic examination of these inclusions by several investigators from 1965 onwards showed that they contained structures similar to paramyxovirus nucleoprotein tubules. Furthermore, using immunofluorescent techniques, antigens of measles virus (a paramyxovirus) were demonstrated in the nucleus and cytoplasm of neurones and glial cells of the cerebral cortex by Connolly and his colleagues in Belfast (See ref. 21).

To date there has been only one report of the transmission of SSPE to experimental animals. Katz and his colleagues (54) inoculated three groups of ferrets intracerebrally with 10% suspensions of brain biopsy material obtained from three different patients with SSPE. Approximately five months after inoculation, animals from each group developed an illness which resembled SSPE both in its symptoms and pathology. Two serial passages of the agent using extracts of diseased ferret brains were achieved while inoculation of ferrets with suspensions of normal human or ferret brain did not produce the disease. Not all the sick animals died, but they all continued to show EEG abnormalities after an apparent clinical recovery. Three ferrets inoculated with a suspension of infected ferret brain which had been incubated with serum from a patient with SSPE remained well, and there was no histological evidence of the disease in one of the animals sacrificed 18 weeks after injection. Electron microscopic examination of brain tissue from sick ferrets did not reveal any virus-like structures and no viruses were recovered using a wide range of tissue cultures. Sera from the affected ferrets did not contain any detectable antibodies to measles virus nor could any specific antigens

be found in the infected brain tissues.  The authors concluded that brains from patients with SSPE contain a transmissible agent causing encephalomyelitis in ferrets, although
they were unable to comment on its nature.  However, since
no further experiments seem to have been reported to date it
is difficult to assess the significance of these observations
so far as SSPE is concerned.

Despite the use of a wide range of experimental animals
and tissue cultures it has proved impossible to isolate any
identifiable infectious virus directly from SSPE brain
material.  However, it was soon discovered that monolayer
cell cultures could be readily grown from such specimens.
Measles antigens were shown to be present in the cultured
cells as well as the original brain tissues, while syncytia
were produced (a characteristic of measles virus infection)
where adjacent cells fuse to form a multinucleated giant cell.
It was from these brain cell cultures that infectious measles
virus was ultimately recovered, on rare occasions from the
supernatant fluids, but most often by co-cultivating or
fusing the antigen-containing cells with a cell line which
was highly permissive for measles virus.  After recovery,
the early passages of the SSPE strains usually grow much more
slowly than do laboratory-adapted strains of measles virus
and it has been suggested that SSPE measles is a specific,
neurotropic variant.  Some investigators maintain that the
SSPE strains are distinct, and there is no doubt that they
show a much greater variation in properties than do laboratory-
adapted strains from patients with acute measles.  On the
other hand, serial passage in permissive cells results, sooner
or later, in the appearance of a growth rate and general
properties similar to those of other laboratory strains.

Indeed, it appears that many of the biophysical characters
of a measles virus strain depend solely on its previous
passage history.   The most widely accepted theory at present,
is that the measles viruses in SSPE are 'defective' and this
will be discussed in detail later.

It is possible that the measles virus could be an
opportunist invader of the damaged brain in SSPE, but the
immunological evidence strongly suggests that it is in fact
the causative organism.   All cases of SSPE have exceptionally
high levels of measles antibodies in both serum and CSF.
The ratio of CSF to serum titers indicates that this is not
due to leakage from the serum but to a local production of
measles antibodies in the CNS.   Furthermore, a proportion
of the antibodies are in the form of IgM which indicates the
continuing synthesis of the structural proteins of measles
virus.   It should be noted here that papovavirus-like
particles, similar to those seen in PML, have also been
visualised by electron microscopy in some cases of SSPE,
but the evidence here suggests that these are indeed
opportunist invaders, although a possible etiological
relationship cannot be completely discounted.

Working from the assumption that the disease process in
SSPE is due to the measles virus infection, two factors
emerge.   Firstly, that the primary infections appear to be
in young children (four years of age or less) and secondly
that the interval before the onset of CNS disease is of the
order of 9 to 13 years.   Since 1968, several cases of SSPE
have been reported in children who had received live atten-
uated measles vaccine between three weeks and three years
prior to onset.   While it cannot be proved that the vaccine
was the cause of the disease, this possibility must always

be kept in mind.    One question, as yet unanswered:  Does the
measles virus become latent or slow in the CNS immediately
following the primary infection, or does it remain latent at
another site and reach the brain after reactivation or alteration?    Using co-cultivation techniques, measles virus has
been isolated from the lymph nodes of two early cases of
SSPE, but not from the lymph nodes of three advanced cases
or five normal controls.    It is therefore possible that the
latent phase is not in the CNS but that the virus is transported there in cells of the lymphocyte or macrophage series.
As measles antigen can be demonstrated in the white cells
from the CSF of patients with SSPE, this is a distinct
possibility.    Replication at non-CNS sites, in particular
in lymphoid cells, appears to be a feature common to all slow
virus infections which we shall discuss later.

Although a few SSPE measles strains are neurotropic
when inoculated intracerebrally into mice and hamsters, this
is not a general property of such strains, nor is it a
property commonly found among strains from typical acute
measles cases.    Nevertheless, it is possible to adapt, by
frequent serial passage in tissue culture, some, if not all,
strains to grow intracerebrally in mice, with or without the
production of disease.    The illness produced in mice by
these neurotropic strains is an acute encephalitis.    It is
important to note here that although measles virus frequently
reaches the CNS in natural infections of man, acute encephalitis occurs as a complication in only a small proportion
of the patients.    The majority of the murine neurotropic
strains of measles virus are strongly cell-associated, with
only relatively small numbers of virions being released from
the infected cells, although relatively large quantities of

cell-bound infectious virus are formed.    Measles virus
isolated from human brain tissue in acute encephalitis also
has similar properties.

Cell cultures, similar to those grown from SSPE brains,
can be grown from measles-infected mouse brains in which the
measles virus also appears to be partially 'defective' (47).
Large quantities  of antigen are produced, but only small
numbers of infectious virions are released into the supernatant fluids.    One property of these persistently infected
cultures is that they are not lysed by the addition of high
titer measles antiserum and complement.    It is apparent,
therefore, that although neurotropic mouse measles produces
a typical acute disease, the virus itself has some of the
properties of measles in SSPE.    While it is very difficult
to relate directly the results of experimental infections in
a foreign host to the natural disease, the ability of several
strains of measles virus to become neurotropic in mice is a
valuable pointer to their ability to become neurotropic in
man.

As stated above, mouse brain cells persistently infected
with measles virus are not affected by specific antiserum.
Rustigian (70) produced a persistent measles virus infection
in Hela cells (a human tumor cell line) from which infectious
virus was released and in which measles antigens could be
demonstrated by immunofluorescence.    When these cells were
cultured in the presence of measles antiserum, a clonal line
was obtained in which only incomplete virus was synthesised
even when the antiserum was removed.

We must now see what conclusions can be drawn from this
evidence.    It is clear that the pathology of the early
lesions is characteristic of a viral encephalitis, while the

relentless progression of the disease to a fatal outcome is
very reminiscent of the other slow virus diseases.   From
the evidence it seems reasonable to conclude that there is
an etiological relationship between SSPE and measles virus
infection.   However the question remains - Is SSPE a 'slow'
or a 'persistent' virus disease?

Although the evidence supports the conclusion that SSPE
is a rare complication of measles virus infection, it is
apparent that the form of the virus which produces SSPE is
very different from that which results in acute measles.
The long interval of up to about ten years between the initial
infection and disease has led to the suggestion that the
measles virus remains latent for much of this time, and is
only reactivated a relatively short time before the onset of
symptoms.   Classical measles is an acute systemic disease,
lasting one to two weeks, sometimes complicated by a typical
acute viral encephalitis.   It is probable that the virus
reaches the CNS in many more children than those in whom an
acute encephalitis develops.   It has therefore been postulated that a latent measles infection is established in at least
a proportion of children, either in the CNS or in some other
site such as the regional lymph nodes, and on reactivation
the measles virus has been altered to a defective form.
The experimental evidence certainly suggests that measles
virus can be altered to a 'defective' state but it is
probably more correct to postulate an alteration to a 'slow'
or 'defective' form in SSPE than to use the term reactivation.
However, this really comes to a matter of semantics and does
not help to decide between the alternative possibilities of a
'slow' or a 'persistent' role for the measles virus.   There
is, nevertheless, one possibly rather telling point in favour

of the supposition that the change involved is one to a 'slow'
virus.    If SSPE is thought of in terms of a 'persistent'
virus - or of a 'latent' virus and reactivation, then there
seems no very good reason why the disease should be so restricted to children and young adolescents and not, so far
as is known, found in older patients.    Further, the neuronal
destruction in SSPE appears to be due to the direct cytopathic effect of the altered measles virus on the cells and
not produced by the action of the immune response to the
measles virus antigens.    If the altered measles infection
were 'persistent' rather than 'slow' we should expect the
virus to have little or no direct effect on the cells, and
any pathology to be due to the immune response.

   We therefore believe that the most probable explanation
of the disease process in SSPE is that the RNA measles virus
is altered in such a way that a 'slow' virus is the outcome.
It has already been concluded that slow viruses will most
probably have DNA cores and that RNA viruses will therefore
have to undergo reverse transcription to a DNA form.    Assuming that such a change occurs to measles virus, then the
sequence of events will resemble that occurring in visna
virus infections.    However, while visna carried its own
reverse transcriptase, measles virus would require the
adventitious presence of such an enzyme system derived from
another source, most probably a co-infecting leukovirus.
Reactivation of a measles-derived DNA provirus followed by
synthesis and release of the original RNA measles virus
would be expected to lead to something similar to an acute
measles encephalitis.    Although the early lesions of SSPE
are characteristic of a viral encephalitis, the later changes
and the very slowness of the disease are quite distinct.

The simple reactivation of a measles proviral DNA cannot therefore be the cause of SSPE.  However because of its complexity we will leave detailed discussion of the possible mechanisms which may be involved in such a change of measles virus to a DNA form until Chapter 14 where slow viruses are considered as a group.

The experimental results also suggest a mechanism by which measles virus may arrive at the point of transformation to a slow form in an infected child.  Following the initial respiratory infection, there is a viremia in which the virus is carried to all parts of the body, including the CNS.  The host responds by producing antibodies and sensitised cells which rapidly bring about the elimination of the bulk of the virus.  We cannot say at what subsequent stage the virus becomes neurotropic, but the experimental results with mice have shown that a prolonged period of cell culture could increase its neurovirulence.  At some point the alteration to the slow form must also occur, but if what we have suggested is correct, then we must ask why does this only happen in such a minute proportion of the children who become infected.  In the first place, it is probable that only a small number of host-virus combinations will be capable of bringing about the necessary sequence of events.  It also seems likely that this will be a chance occurrence, depending on the properties of the infecting virus, its compatibility with the host-cell genome the overall pattern of the immune response of the host and, if our hypothesis is correct, the presence of reverse transcriptase.  Measles virus itself is known to suppress cell-mediated immunity, and this introduces a further variable.  Any hypothesis concerning SSPE must contain some 'chance' element to explain why only one of the pair of identical twins who were simultaneously infected with what was presumably the same strain of measles virus in early childhood later developed the disease while the other remained completely well.

At this point it should be remembered that measles virus belongs to a sub-group of closely related paramyxoviruses which includes canine distemper and rinderpest of cattle. Distemper virus (CDV) causes a severe respiratory illness in dogs, sometimes accompanied by an acute meningo-encephalitis. Like measles, it is believed that CDV enters the CNS in the majority of infected dogs, whether or not symptoms develop. In addition a demyelinating encephalomyelitis occurs as a late complication in a proportion of dogs which recover from the acute illness.   The CNS signs appear several weeks or even months after recovery from the acute disease and the lesions resemble experimental allergic encephalomyelitis. Experimentally the late onset diseases can be induced in gnotobiotic dogs following an incubation period of five to six weeks.   Only one strain of CDV will regularly produce a fatal encephalomyelitis following intracerebral inoculation, although demyelination, and more rarely death, may occur after inoculation by other routes or with other strains of virus.   In a recent review Koestner and his colleagues (56) suggest that the demyelination is virus induced and is dependent upon the presence of certain mutant strains of CDV. These mutants have not yet been fully characterised, but are believed to be better able to persist in brain than 'typical' strains.   They are also thought to be able to trigger an anti-myelin response possibly due to membrane alteration in glial cells independent of viral maturation.   Koestner concluded with the theory that anti-myelin antibodies

probably amplify the virus-induced membrane lesions although
the role of sensitised lymphocytes has not been established.
As the CDV - late onset encephalomyelitis system shows some
similarities to the measles virus - SSPE system it may prove
to be a useful model.

CHAPTER XI


MULTIPLE SCLEROSIS


Although the evidence in favour of a viral etiology for
multiple sclerosis (MS) is circumstantial, it is appropriate
to discuss it at this point as much of the current information
implicates measles virus as the most likely causative agent.
Multiple sclerosis is the archetype of demyelinating diseases.
It occurs in several clinical forms and is often difficult to
differentiate from other syndromes except at autopsy.

The pathology of the brain in MS is characterised by
areas or plaques, of demyelination.   The plaques may be
completely demyelinated, or made up of concentric rings of
demyelination alternating with rings showing relative preser-
vation of the myelin sheaths.   The axis cylinders within the
plaques are spared and may remain normal for long periods,
although degeneration ultimately occurs.   The lesions are
centred round small blood vessels and are spread throughout


135

the nervous system in both space and time.    In acute lesions
a perivascular inflammatory infiltration similar to that seen
in acute viral encephalitis is found, while hypertrophy of
astroglial cells appears early and persists throughout the
disease.    The presence of inclusion bodies typical of
measles virus infection has been reported by J. M. Adams,
but this interpretation of the histology is disputed by
other workers (see ref. 41).    The majority of reports on
the electron microscopy of MS brain have failed to add
significantly to our knowledge of the disease, although
recently it has been claimed that structures typical of
paramyxovirus nucleoprotein tubules are present in the
tissues.

The epidemiology of MS has received considerable attention.    Geographically the world can be divided into zones
of high and low risk for the acquisition of the disease.
Analysis of the epidemiological data especially concerning
migrations between zones, indicates that MS has an infectious
etiology, and that the causative agent is acquired when the
patient is around the age of puberty.    On the other hand,
an increase in CSF gamma-globulins has led to suggestions
that the disease is primarily an 'autoimmune' process.    As
might be expected it has also been suggested that MS is a
composite disease, consisting of an infectious process which
produces the acute form, followed by an autoimmune response
resulting from host reaction to the infection process,
which itself produces the chronic form.    There is, of course,
no reason why both processes should not be involved, either
simultaneously or sequentially, in which case the disease
would have many of the features of a persistent infection.
However, we shall not consider this further here, but con-

centrate on the evidence associating known virus infections
with MS.

Several groups of workers in Europe and America have
compared the levels of viral antibodies in the serum of MS
patients with the levels in normal individuals or in patients
with other neurological disorders.    The majority of investigators have shown that the mean levels of measles antibodies
are higher in MS patients than in controls.    In some series,
antibody levels to herpes simplex virus were also elevated,
but in general, measles virus is the only one in which the
association has been found with a reasonable degree of consis-
tency.    The presence of measles antibodies in the CSF has
also been measured in some series and again they are elevated
in patients with MS, although not to the same degree as in
cases of SSPE.    By and large the bulk of the CSF measles
antibodies are directed against the internal nucleoprotein
of the virus and are detected by complement fixation (CF)
tests, although those directed against the haemagglutinin
(HI antibodies), a component of the viral coat, are sometimes
found.    These studies suggest that the antibodies in individual CSF specimens are directed against only one viral
component antigen.    An examination of serum specimens from
43 patients with active MS showed the presence of measles
IgM in four and mumps IgM in two patients.    In one case each,
mumps IgM and measles IgM appeared to have persisted for at
least two and a half years.    In a comparable group of 43
patients with other nervous system diseases, measles IgM was
found in only one serum, while among 43 normal control
patients no measles or mumps IgM was found.    The serological
results therefore indicate the presence of a persistent
infection of the CNS of MS patients by measles or perhaps

some other paramyxovirus.    The recovery of an infectious
paramyxovirus has in fact been reported from the brains of
two MS cases.    Parainfluenza type 1, which is antigenically
related to mumps virus, was recovered from the first case by
the use of a cell fusion technique, and measles was isolated
from the second by co-cultivation.

        Taken in conjunction with the clinical and epidemiological
data, the persistence of paramyxovirus antibodies in a proportion of MS cases suggests, although less clearly than in
SSPE, that the disease may also result from a change in the
form of the original paramyxovirus.    There is, of course
the obvious possibility that measles (or any other paramyxovirus) may be an opportunist invader and have no etiological
significance.    However if this is not the case an explanation of the phenomenon must be sought, particularly bearing
in mind that if a change in measles results in SSPE, how
might MS arise as a more common disease in the same way?
The suggestion has already been made that the essential step
in the development of SSPE is a reverse transcription of the
original measles RNA to a DNA form.    The serological data
coupled with the ability to recover infectious measles virus
from the infected brain tissues in SSPE indicates that the
putative DNA provirus must be a reasonably complete and
accurate copy of the original RNA.    It is obvious that
accurate and complete reverse transcription of the RNA
normally occurs with leukoviruses which carry their own
enzymes, but it is by no means certain that reverse transcription by an adventitious enzyme would necessarily be so
complete or accurate.    It is therefore possible that an
incomplete or inaccurate reverse transcription of measles
(or other paramyxovirus) RNA could result in a 'defective'

DNA provirus which is the cause of MS.   In the paramyxovirus
(unlike the leukoviruses) the messenger RNA strand is not the
virion strand and failure to transcribe either the virion
strand or the RNA replicase coded in the viral nucleic acid
would completely prevent the formation of measles virions.
It would appear that the scope for the production of a defective provirus is almost unlimited (providing it happens at
all).   Further, in the previous chapter it was noted that
measles virus is closely related to canine distemper virus
and it could be postulated that MS might arise by reverse
transcription not of measles RNA but of canine distemper RNA.
There are just about as many theories concerning the role of
measles and other factors in the etiology of MS as there are
individuals working on the disease, and the interested
reader is referred to the Symposium Proceedings edited by
Field et al. (41).

Before leaving MS two other reports must be mentioned.
Transmission of a scrapie-like disease to sheep and mice
from one specimen of MS brain has been claimed (40) but has
not yet been repeated.

In 1972 reports from Carp and his group (14,60) appeared
of a decreased percentage of polymorphonuclear neutrophils
(PMN) in mouse peripheral blood following the injection of
either MS material, or scrapie material from infected mice
or sheep, but not after normal tissue injection.   The
factor(s) were then shown to be transmissible in mice and to
reach incredibly high titers in the brain (of the order of
$10^{12}$ $ID_{50}$ in 0.03ml of 20% brain homogenate).   With MS
material at least, the factor causing the changes in PMN
counts was detectable between 12 hrs and $8\frac{1}{2}$ months after
inoculation.   Subsequently a contrary report has appeared

(13) and two confirmatory reports, one on scrapie (27) and
one on MS material (57).   It is clear from the various
publications that the assay system (PMN counts) is unreliable
and suffers from many problems such as an inherent base line
instability, and this makes it difficult at present to accept
the whole package unreservedly.   However the best assessment
one can make at the time of writing is that Carp is correct
in supposing that there is a rapidly replicating persistent
agent occurring in both MS patients and scrapie infected
animals.   If this is so the question then arises as to the
relationship between the Carp agent or agents and these two
diseases.   In the first place it is quite clear as Carp
himself has pointed out, that the Carp and scrapie agents
must be separate and distinct, since Carp agent occurs in
brain at a titer several logs higher than the scrapie agent.
The latter can therefore be diluted out, and mice thus
inoculated with Carp agent alone have shown no signs of
scrapie over a prolonged period.   Although it is not at
present entirely clear whether Carp agent occurs in high
titer in serum as well as in brain, it obviously has striking
similarities - in titer and persistence - to the Riley (LDH)
virus, which in fact has also been found associated (as a
contaminant) with a scrapie mouse colony (8).   Although again
it is clear that the Carp and LDH agents must be different,
there is no reason to suppose that the LDH agent is the only
one of its type - and in fact its own discovery was highly
fortuitous.   If Carp agent were associated only with scrapie
then an LDH type contaminant would be the most likely explanation.   However - again assuming the validity of the experimental results - it is very difficult to explain its association with material from MS patients in this way.   Although

by analogy with scrapie it would also seem highly unlikely
that Carp agent is the cause of MS, it may well be associated
in some direct manner with the actual etiological agent.    If
this is correct it would also seem probable that scrapie
'Carp' and MS 'Carp' although similar are not one and the
same.    However a further possibility concerning the relationship between Carp agent and MS will be discussed later in
this volume.

The only summary which can be made at present is that
the circumstantial evidence suggesting an infectious etiology
for MS is matched by the number of claims for potential
causative agents.    Only time and further investigation will
enable the significance of the present data to be assessed.

CHAPTER XII

FACTORS INFLUENCING THE INCUBATION PERIOD OF SLOW VIRUSES

There are a number of factors which influence the overall time from infection to onset of symptoms but again most
of the experimental information relating to slow viruses is
derived from studies on the scrapie agent.

GENETIC FACTORS

Following inoculation with scrapie agent, mice, rats
and goats show an almost complete incidence of the disease
whereas a proportion of sheep, the natural host, is resistant. Strains of sheep vary considerably in their susceptibility and, as has been said, this appears to reflect the
operation of genetic factors. Sheep may, in fact, be bred
for the development of scrapie resistance and it seems

possible, in principle at least, that the disease could be eradicated by proper selection.

By far the most significant information on the inter-action of genetic factors and scrapie has come from the work of Dickinson and his group in Edinburgh (25, 26). They have isolated a number of different strains of mouse scrapie agent which were characterisable by differences in the distribution and morphological patterns of the brain lesions. The strains fell into two groups on the basis of the lengths of their incubation periods in two strains of mice. Evidence was then obtained that the control of the length of the incubation period was vested in a single gene, the "sinc" gene, which consisted of two alleles referred to as s7 and p7. The variations in the length of incubation period brought about by the various combinations of alleles and agents were very striking. For example, in C57 mice, homozygous for the s7 allele, the average incubation period for the ME7 strain of scrapie agent was about 160 days, and for the 22A strain about 450 days. In VM mice, homozygous for the p7 allele, the figures were 200 days for 22A and 320 days for ME7, so that in this strain the respective lengths of the incubation period were reversed. Recalling what has been said concern-ing the relative constancy of the time course of scrapie and other slow virus diseases, it may be re-emphasised that the individual results making up each of these different incuba-tion periods were concentrated into a narrow time band. There seem to be no really comparable results with other viruses and so it is not possible to say at present whether scrapie is unique in this respect, or whether such genetic influences extend to other slow agents or indeed to viruses as a whole. There does not even seem to be any obvious explanation of the mechanism as far as scrapie is concerned. One could talk generally in terms of the regulation of gene expression and genetic control of host systems such as those responsible for synthesis of macromolecules, repression and derepression, or even of individual enzyme reactions, but this adds very little to our understanding of the mechanism. It is also tempting to say that genetic control would link very well with the supposition that slow virus DNA is incorporated into the host genomes, but again this would be rather an ad hoc correlation.

The variations in the incubation period of scrapie in mice resulting from genetic factors give some support to the view that the variations seen in sheep, and the failure of a proportion of some strains to develop the disease at all, are similarly due to variations in genetic make up.    It would therefore seem reasonable to suggest that in some circumstances the reason for failure to develop scrapie is that the onset of the disease has been delayed beyond the lifespan of the animal (24).    This underlines the overlapping of the slow and latent groups of viruses.    However, conclusions of this nature involving the lifespan of animals must be treated with some caution, since, for example, very few sheep are allowed to live long enough to die naturally.    In this case the failure of some to develop scrapie may therefore be more apparent than real.


HOST ADAPTATION


The scrapie agent, in common with other viruses, goes through a process of 'adaptation' to a new host characterised by a progressive shortening of the incubation period.    When

mice are inoculated with preparations of scrapie sheep brain
it may take 12 months or more before unmistakable clinical
disease develops, while five years was required for transmission to a single cynamolgus monkey (although in squirrel
monkeys the incubation time was only 14 months (42).   Thus,
the initial transfer of slow virus diseases from species to
species may be as great an exercise in patience as in
scientific skill and where the attempt is from a long-lived
species (e.g. man) to short-lived laboratory animals it is
not difficult to see how easily time can run out before
anything happens.   Consequently attempts to transmit multiple
sclerosis, for example, to animals may have failed for this
reason rather than because of any inherent incompatibility.
However, once scrapie has developed in mice after transfer
from sheep, successive passages reduce the time span progressively, until the time taken from inoculation to death is
about six months.

Could man become infected with scrapie?  This possibility has always been present, but the successful transmission
of the disease to primates raises the question in a much more
acute form.   In particular, two groups of people could be
considered as being at risk.   Firstly the comparatively
small group of laboratory workers carrying out research on
the disease, some of whom have handled infected tissues over
a very long period of time.   So far fortunately there is no
clear evidence than any have succumbed to any recognisable
central nervous system disease.   Secondly a very much larger
group of people who almost inevitably have eaten scrapie
infected sheep at some time.   Although oven roasting of meat
from a scrapie sheep (in which the titre of scrapie agent is
low anyway) would probably destroy nearly all of it, sheep

brain lightly poached in milk has been considered a delicacy
in certain areas such as parts of the North of England.   Such
treatment of brain from a scrapie-infected sheep would almost
certainly result in the consumption of relatively large
amounts of infective agent.   Although there is no way of
telling whether one or other of the obscure CNS diseases of
man may actually be 'scrapie' the possibility cannot now be
dismissed lightly.


EFFECT OF SIZE OF INOCULUM


    It is a well known phenomenon, with all viruses, that
the time taken for disease to develop, or for peak virus
titer to be reached, depends on the number of infective doses
present in the original inoculum.   There are some obvious
reasons for this.   For example within limits, the larger the
dose, the larger is the number of cells which will be infected
initially, and so fewer replication cycles are required to
reach the final state.   The initial proportion of infected
to non-infected cells may also influence the rate of interferon and antibody production.   Dickinson's group have
recently published data on the effect on the incubation period
in mice (to the appearance of clinical disease) of varying
the initial intracerebral inoculum of scrapie from one to $10^5$
infectious doses.   The resulting incubation periods lay on a
smooth curve and varied between 400 and 200 days at the
extreme (23).   These data do not tell us how the increased
time span is divided between the latent period before replication begins, and the time taken for the replication period.
However, there seems no reason why, once a reasonable titer
has been attained, there should from then on be any marked

difference in replication rate.   If this is so then the
total time during which replication is occurring can only be
increased by the length of time required for a small inoculum
to reach the starting point of a large one.   The best guess
is that the increase in incubation period resulting from
reducing the inoculum is divided between latent period and
replication period in such a way that the approximate relationship between the two is maintained.


ARTIFICIAL DELAY

It is possible to extend the latent period of normally
fast viruses by artificial means, for example, by putting the
host into a state of low metabolic activity.   When garter
snakes are infected with Western Equine encephalitis virus
and then hibernated, virus replication does not occur until
the appropriate time after the reptile is removed from
hibernation.   The explanation of the prolonged latent period
in this case is probably that when the host as a whole is
synthesising macromolecules at a very low rate, which presumably is the situation during hibernation, then the virus
cannot induce its own replication.   It is important to
realise that situations such as this differ fundamentally
from the slow virus pattern as the next section explains.


RELATIONSHIP BETWEEN THE LATENT PERIOD AND REPLICATION PHASE

In general, the viral replication phase after infection
of individual or synchronously related cells follows an
approximately sigmoid curve.   It can only be approximately

sigmoid because the factors operating at the "initiation"
end are different from those at the "termination" end.    The
central part of the curve is probably exponential, corresponding to a log growth phase.    The latent phase preceeds
and leads into the replication phase and, as already stated,
in the case of a typical virus the replication phase is
terminated by the production of interferon and the immune
response.    In the case of Riley virus the whole curve has
been determined experimentally in mice and is given in Figure
3.    As shown in the figure the latent period, during which
there is only a very small titer of virus in the plasma,
occupies approximately six hours and the total time to peak
titer is about 16 hours.    Thus the incubation period is
divided approximately in the ratio  2:3 of latent period:
replication phase.    Incidentally and as remarked before, in
the final stage of decline the titer of Riley virus does not
return to zero, but to a lower persistent level - the hallmark of a persistent virus infection.

     The latent period itself is also a combination of at
least two stages when the number of susceptible cells is very
much larger than the infecting dose.    As soon as the virus
enters its host cell and becomes uncoated its infectivity is
virtually zero because of the loss of infective efficiency
which is associated with naked nucleic acid.    At this stage
then, the virus may be considered as having entered an
"eclipse" phase, in that it is undetectable.    Fast viruses
then rapidly enter their assembly and maturation stage which
results in the production and release of new infectious
virions from the cell.    Although infectious virus may then
be detectable this second phase may be regarded as part of
the latent period because most of the new virions must be

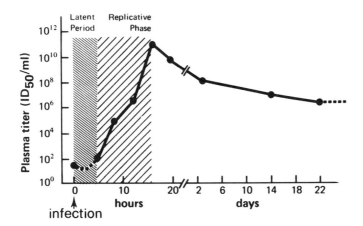

Fig. 3
Change in plasma titer of mouse lactate dehydrogenase — elevating virus
after infection of the host animal. The approximate lengths of the latent
and replicative phases are indicated. After reaching peak titer the level in
the plasma falls more slowly and persists indefinitely at around $10^6$ $ID_{50}$
units/ml.
*(After Adams and Bowman, (5))*

used to infect adjacent cells if the infection is to progress. After each new cycle of infection the invading virus disappears in order to begin the whole process over again.    The latent period, during which infective virus is virtually absent, will not end therefore until a sufficient number of new virions is produced to create a surplus resulting in an increasing titer.

Similar data on the time taken by the various stages does not seem to be available for most viruses, but such evidence as there is suggests again an approximately 2:3 ratio of latent period to replication phase.    Further, where the conditions are appropriately controlled, the pattern in vitro is also similar.    For example - the latent period of the togavirus hemorrhagic fevers is about five days before the onset of illness associated with the appearance of a viremia. The acute stage of the illness lasts for five to ten days and the viremia does not persist beyond this stage.    In human tissue cultures, poliovirus has a latent period of three to four hours followed by a replication phase of four to six hours.    A less rapid cycle occurs in monkey kidney cells infected with SV40 virus.    Incorporation of precursors into viral DNA begins about 15 hours after inoculation and reaches a maximum after 30 hours, while the peak of plaque forming virus is reached by about 50 hours.    These examples all seem very clear cut and reasonable.    However what is perhaps surprising is that when the available information concerning the scrapie agent is looked at in the same way it also fits the same pattern, i.e. as already stated, a relatively fast strain of mouse scrapie is associated with a latent period of about 8-10 weeks and a replication phase of about 12-15 weeks.    Results with scrapie in spleen, where

the incubation period is shorter, also show an approximately
2:3 ratio of latent period:replication phase.   It may be
pointed out that with an agent such as scrapie, where the
time scale of the process is so extended, it is more difficult to assess accurately either the point of peak titer, or
that delineating the changeover from latent to replication
phase.   However, considering the variations in types of
virus, host tissues in vivo, and host cells in vitro, the
correlation between the ratios of latent period and replication phase appears remarkably good.

   It seems probable that this correlation is, in fact,
built in to the system by the parameters governing the
overall growth rates of the individual viruses.   As has
been indicated, the steps following the entry of a virion
into the first host cell are as follows:-

|  | (i) | (ii) | (iii) |
|---|---|---|---|
| Virion → | Host cell → | Uncoating → | Nucleic acid com- → ponent makes mess- enger and templates for synthesis of viral nucleic acid and protein |

|  | (iv) |  | (v) |  | (vi) |
|---|---|---|---|---|---|
| New virions produced | → | New virions re- leased to infect other cells | → |  | Titer begins to → build up when more virions are produced than are needed for spreading the infec- tion |

   Steps (ii) and (iii) represent the 'eclipse' phase,
steps (ii) through (v) the overall 'latent' phase, and step
(vi) the beginning of the replication phase.   It seems
clear that the rate of production of new virions will be
reflected in the rate at which steps (v) and (vi) can occur

and it is not unreasonable to suggest that this would automatically produce a temporal relationship between the two
phases (latent and replicative) which would hold over wide
rate variations.

If this interpretation is correct, then the fact that
the scrapie agent follows a pattern similar to that of the
fast viruses is further evidence that the slow agents are
part of the total virus spectrum.    It also underlines the
essential difference between 'slowness' and 'latency' - in
the latter the replication rate before activation is zero or
limited to keeping pace with the host genome during cell
division.    Latent viruses do not replicate in the normal
sense until activation occurs and then the process proceeds
at a rate which bears no relation to the period of latency.

CHAPTER XIII

SLOW VIRUSES AS A GROUP

The common behaviour of the slow viruses in relation to the lack of an effective immune or interferon response by the infected host has already been discussed at length.  In this sense, at least, they do seem to form a group which to some extent differentiates them from most other viruses.  In this chapter we shall consider how far they may be similarly grouped together on the basis of other characteristics.

The comment has often been made that the major part of our fragmentary knowledge of the nature and properties of the slow growing viruses has been derived from studies on scrapie.  Unfortunately, not only have the unusual proper- ties of the scrapie agent tended to obscure its true nature, but at present we really do not know how far they are shared by slow viruses as a whole.  However, the recent successes in transmitting the other agents of the spongiform enceph-

alopathy group to experimental animals have allowed at least
a provisional comparison to be made of their properties in
relation to those of the scrapie agent.   In fact, at the
time of writing, the evidence supports the view that the
agents responsible for this group of diseases do resemble
each other in their nature and properties.   Thus in all
probability the scrapie agent is not unique, as was thought
to be the case until recently.   It also seems clear that
the properties of the spongiform encephalopathy group of
agents differ in many ways from those of visna-maedi virus
or of the PML papovavirus.   Nevertheless, from the biological standpoint all the slow viruses seem to have much in
common, both as a group, and when considered in relation to
the faster classical viruses.   Further, the evidence is
well established for the presence of nucleic acid as the
genetic material in the visna-maedi and PML agents and indeed
in SSPE, with the proviso that we do not know for certain
what the steps are which connect the RNA of measles virus
with the rare SSPE disease.   In our opinion then the slow
infective agents can be considered as a sub-group (possibly
sub-divided again into the spongiform encephalopathies and
others) falling within the classical virus definition as
part of the total virus spectrum.

    We realise, of course, that if the conclusion that the
scrapie agent is based on nucleic acid is incorrect, then it
will not be possible to treat the slow infective agents as a
single group.   Indeed in this case the nature of the whole
spongiform encephalopathy group of agents might also have to
be rethought.   It would also follow that such a conclusion
would render meaningless much of the attempt made so far in
this volume to relate the slow virus pattern as a whole to

the properties and metabolism of the nucleic acids.    However,
the balance of the evidence supports the view that all the
slow agents are, or will be shown to be, nucleic acid based.
Consequently the enquiry into their nature and properties will
continue on that assumption.

From a consideration of general biochemical principles
we had reached the tentative conclusion that DNA would be a
more suitable core for a slow virus than RNA.    The suita-
bility of DNA was based on the view that RNA synthesis seems
geared to rapidity, and it would be too difficult to slow
down any of the normally fast synthetic reactions sufficiently to produce the required slow, steady, rate of production,
while still retaining the necessary control.    Although this
conclusion seems reasonable on general grounds, it may be
criticised as being little better than an educated guess.
However, having considered the biology and the disease-
producing characteristics of the slow viruses in some
detail, it is now possible to make some rather more direct
suggestions on the results which might be expected to occur
if one of the synthetic reactions or assembly steps proceeded
at a drastically reduced rate necessary in a slow virus
disease.    The problem of doing this while still retaining
the cohesiveness of the overall system, has already been
touched on, and it would seem reasonable to suppose that the
rate of the particular reaction or step would have to be
controlled within very narrow limits.    If we take, as an
example, a single reaction limiting the rate of production
of viral RNA - which is so susceptible to degradation - the
rate of synthesis would seem very liable to dip below that
necessary to maintain a net increase.    This would probably
end in the abortion of the infection.    If the synthetic

rate were marginally too fast, the most likely result would
be a snowballing of production and a fairly rapid infection.
While perhaps less susceptible to degradation, similar problems seem likely to arise if the postulated rate limiting
step were associated with the production of capsid or coat
protein, or of viral DNA as long as it remained 'free' within
the cell.   Although theoretically it might be possible to
adjust the overall reaction rate in this way to fit the slow
virus pattern it seems inescapable that in the event the
balance between 'go' and 'no go' or between 'slow go' and
'fast go' would rest on a knife edge.   Since between individual animals there are inherent variations in all enzyme
levels, reaction rates, and also no doubt rates of assembly
of virus components, one would be led to the logical conclusion that the infection of groups of animals with slow
viruses would produce extremely variable results, both in
terms of the time taken between inoculation and onset of
disease or death, and in the proportion of animals developing
the disease at all.   It is also probable that the variation
in response of individual animals would be significantly
increased by varying the infecting dose.   At present the
best experimental system against which these conclusions can
be compared is that of the development of scrapie in mice.
As has been indicated, when a given scrapie dose is inoculated
into even a relatively heterogenous strain of mice, not only
is infection universal, but the time required for the onset
of clinical signs and death is relatively constant.   Further,
although there is a greater spread in the individual incubation periods when lower infective doses are used, the effect
is not great, and is in similar proportion to the spread
shown by fast viruses in the same circumstances.   Particularly

in genetically homogeneous strains, the relationship between
incubation period and infecting dose is so consistent that
many scrapie workers use the time interval between inoculation
and death as a method of estimating the virus titer of the
inocula.    Although comparatively few studies have been made
on other slow virus diseases, the recent evidence concerning
the transmissability of the other agents of the spongiform
encephalopathy group suggests that this pattern of almost
universal takes after proper inoculation and a relatively
constant time course of the disease is similar.    Far from
being a 'knife edge' process therefore, the pattern of slow
virus diseases suggests a constant progression, quite accurately under the control of some 'biological clock' which
regulates the whole inexorable process from its beginning
to its normally fatal end. In our view these considerations
suggest that the slow virus replication and disease process
is effected not by some chance or random slowness of one or
more steps in relation to the rest, but by an integrated and
controlled slowing of the whole sequence.    If this is so
then it follows, of course, that virtually all the reactions
involved must be operating at rates far below their full
potential.

Perhaps at this point a clarification should be made of
the relationship between rates of nucleic acid synthesis
which (a) occur in tissues, and (b) are associated with viral
replication.    Various comments have been made about rates of
replication of slow and fast viruses, rates of tissue growth
and of DNA synthesis relative to RNA synthesis in tissues.
If however a comparison is made between rates of DNA synthesis
which occur in viruses and tissues, the results are perhaps
somewhat unexpected.

In the mouse, for example, a fast growing tumor will
double its weight every 3 days, and mouse fetal tissue grows
similarly.    Cells of the mouse reticulo-endothelial system
divide even more rapidly with a doubling time of about 36
hours.    These figures of course also mirror the average
rates of DNA synthesis.    However, since the cells involved
are only synthesising DNA for about a third of their division
time, the average rate is related to the actual rate by the
same factor whereas in a viral system the average rate is
probably close to the true rate.    Cell division in cancer or
fetal tissue involves the synthesis of comparatively large
quantities of DNA and in many tumors the DNA may make up 1%
or more of the total tissue weight.    DNA viruses on the
other hand normally synthesise DNA far more rapidly, but the
total amount involved is small in comparison.    Probably no
DNA virus replicates in mammalian cells as rapidly as the
Riley (RNA) agent with its doubling time of 20 min. or so,
but a doubling time of 60 min. can be achieved by the fastest
of them.    In contrast Fig. 4 shows an approximate picture
of the replication of a fast strain of scrapie in various
tissues in its host mouse.    The brain titer rises by about
8 logs in 12 weeks, corresponding to a doubling time of
about 4 days.    As stated previously, spleen titer begins to
increase earlier and has reached a plateau at about the time
when the brain titer starts to rise.    The replication is
faster than in brain with a doubling time of about 24-36
hours.    Slower replicating strains of scrapie in mice, scrapie in sheep and the human spongiform agents will have brain
agent doubling times ranging from about 6 to perhaps as long
as 30 days or more in exceptional cases.
    To summarise, the doubling times of normal mammalian

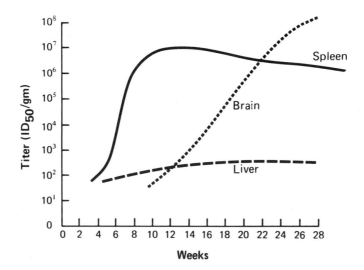

Fıg. 4
Probable course of development of scrapie infective agent titer in
representative mouse tissues after the intracerebral inoculation of
a small number of infective particles  $10^3$  ID/50.
*Data based on the results of several authors.*

tissues spread over the very wide range of about 36 hrs. to
infinity.   However while fast growing tumors again have a
doubling time of 36 hrs. or so, there must be very few with
a doubling time exceeding 50 days.   Because of the approximate parallelism between weight increase and net DNA synthesis the same pattern holds for DNA.   Consequently, bearing in mind the difference between 'average' and 'true'
rates of DNA synthesis, the calculations show that although
slow virus replication rates are slow by comparison with
classical viruses, broadly speaking they fall within the
range of tumor DNA synthetic rates.   The situation in
regard to tissue RNA synthesis is more complex because
although obviously net RNA synthesis must also parallel tissue
growth rates, as already mentioned there is a very rapid
turnover (i.e. synthesis + degradation) of some RNA types,
even in tissues such as the CNS with a virtually zero rate
of either DNA synthesis or turnover.   This rapid turnover
makes it difficult to estimate the acutal rates at which RNA
is synthesised in tissues.   Clearly however the range of
synthetic rates of say nuclear RNA is far narrower than that
of DNA, and probably the average will fall somewhere near
the fast end of the slow virus range.

What sort of restraint then does a tissue appear to be
able to exert in practice on, say, scrapie DNA replication?
So far as the CNS is concerned estimates of scrapie replication times have been given and these obviously vary considerably.   The known governing factors seem to be (a) strain
of agent, (b) strain differences within species, (c) species
of animal - scrapie in sheep or goats having a longer incubation period than in rats or mice.   It seems unlikely (though
not impossible) that central nervous system DNA replication

rates would vary to this extent in the various strains and
species of animals:   indeed metabolic stability of such DNA
seems a characteristic of all mammals.   Consequently if our
suggestion is correct, restraint on scrapie DNA replication
imposed by CNS tissue must operate in the presence of other,
as yet unknown factors which are able to influence the overall rate.   It is also clear, however that the scrapie agent
is only able to replicate two or three times as fast in the
rapidly dividing reticulo endothelial (RE) tissues as it
does in the CNS.   Thus despite the (presumably) much more
severe restraint on DNA replication in the CNS, this tissue
is only able to hold back scrapie multiplication to a
relatively small additional extent.   However what may be
important is that the rate of scrapie replication, even in
the rapidly dividing RE tissue, is still slow compared with
that of the average fast virus.   This is consistent with
the thesis that slow virus replication is restrained by its
host tissue, instead of cutting loose to a greater or lesser
extent as the fast viruses do.

Broadly speaking then slow virus replication occurs over
the same range of rates as does neoplastic cell DNA.   This
indirectly supports the analogy between slow viruses and
neoplastic growth which has already been made and reinforces
the suggestion that slow viruses are based on DNA, with a
similarly regulated and progressive rate of net synthesis
which is very slow in relation to the common viruses but
which cannot be turned off by normal regulatory mechanisms.
How then does this come about?   To digress for a moment,
it is well known that bacteria, for example, will ingest or
take up DNA from outside themselves, and many studies have
been made on the subsequent fate of the DNA.   It can enter

the cells, among other ways, by direct uptake, by infection
with phage or other agents, or by conjugation.   The DNA may
then survive and multiply;  it may be degraded by host enzyme
systems (a process known as 'restriction');  it may be modified - for example methylated by host methylase enzymes - or,
and for our purposes most importantly, it may enter and
become part of the host genome.   It is this last possibility
which we believe to be the key to the slow virus pattern.

In the case of bacteria, such entry of phage DNA into
the host genome is referred to as 'lysogeny'.   When several
years ago this phenomenon was first discovered and investigated, too much emphasis was placed, and too many hopes
pinned, on the proposition that the phage - bacterial system
would be closely analogous to that of the virus - vertebrate
host.   The general problems which have arisen from this concept and the resulting swing to what is probably too far in
the opposite direction do not come within the scope of this
volume.   However in this particular instance the assimilation
of phage into bacterial host-cell DNA does seem to have
analogies to the phenomenon of viral latency (and transformation) in vertebrate cells.   In both bacterial and vertebrate
systems latent phage or virus can be reactivated to give a
fast and lytic infection.   In bacteria the reactivation process is currently being studied in relation to genetics, and
a considerable amount of information concerning the regulatory mechanisms has already been uncovered.   How far the
results from bacterial genetics are applicable to mammalian
and other vertebrate systems is not clear, but it would
seem likely that the broad outlines are similar.   However,
as the entry of viral DNA into the mammalian cell genome may
result in latency or transformation, then obviously if it is

also to be the key to the slow virus pattern a further factor
must be involved to distinguish 'slowness' from both 'transformation' and 'latency' or 'latency' followed by reactivation.

The phenomenon of cell 'take over' discussed previously
applies to both DNA and RNA viruses, although precisely what
'information' is carried by a virus, which enables it to
override cell mechanisms in this way, is not known.   In this
case there is an analogy between fast viruses and fast
growing tumors in that both may well synthesise DNA either
at rates or in amounts which really are limited by the
capacity of the synthetic mechanisms, or the availability of
precursors.   A major qualitative difference is that in the
case of viruses the DNA synthesised is viral DNA, while in
tumors the product is something at least similar to normal
host DNA, and the production is synchronously related to cell
division.   We have already suggested that a reduced 'take
over' ability would lead to slower viral replication.
Proceeding then on these lines, it seems reasonable to
suggest that in some cases viral DNA which has an even further
reduced 'take over' ability may associate with the host genome, but subsequently rather than entering into a state of
true latency, its replication may be restrained to a rate
which is related to that of host cell DNA.

Tentatively therefore, we propose that the essence of
a slow virus lies in the following criteria:-

1)    It is based on DNA.
2)    It has a very limited ability to take over and direct
      the metabolic activity of its host cells, and as a
      consequence the viral genome becomes associated with
      the host genome.
3)    Its replicative ability is not lost, but once in situ

the viral DNA is subjected to constraints on its replication similar to those exerted on host DNA and these
may be very severe in adult mammalian cells.   Further,
that through the viral DNA, these constraints are
passed on to the other viral components so that their
rate of production is kept in step.

It would follow from this that although latent viruses
could be defined in similar terms, by extrapolation of section 3 they would, under normal circumstances, be entirely
constrained within their host cells, and to all intents and
purposes be unable to break the deadlock without assistance.
Consequently there would be no very sharp dividing line
between the two groups.

In certain circumstances it is normal to speak of the
viral DNA as "integrating" into the host genome.   However
this description tends to be used in a very general way
without giving any clear definition of what is involved.
For the moment, therefore we have refrained from using the
term "integrate" until we have considered what is involved
in more detail.   It seems clear that in certain circumstances an external DNA may 'integrate' with host cell chromosomal material in such a way that to all intents and purposes it becomes a structural unit.   While it remains in
this type of association, replication will probably only
occur if and when chromosomal DNA as a whole replicates -
normally as a step in cell division.   In this way the new
DNA also becomes part of the daughter cell chromosomes.
This appears to be the situation in cells which have been
transformed by adenoviruses, papovaviruses and leukoviruses,
although in the latter case it is of course the proviral DNA
which integrates.   However, 'foreign' DNA must, to a greater

or lesser extent, have a potentiality for escaping from its chromosomal niche. Consequently, the events following this type of structural integration will depend, among other things, on the extent to which the integration can be reversed.

There is however another form of integration, which occurs with the herpes viruses and some bacteriophage, in which the viral DNA integrates in a way which can be described as primarily "metabolic" rather than structural. It is this type of "integration" which we consider to be much more likely in the case of slow virus nucleic acid cores. Such a non-structural type of association will probably provide something less in the way of protection, but more in the way of independent replicative capacity.

Would this mean that RNA viruses can never be 'slow' or 'latent'? The evidence so far presented has suggested that they cannot, and further there seems no way in which RNA per se can take refuge in the host cell genome as can DNA. However, the original dogma of molecular biology laid perhaps too much stress on the view that all cellular information flowed from DNA into RNA into protein, but never in the reverse direction. Basically there is no great difference between the structures of DNA and RNA, and even on general grounds it would not seem surprising that information in RNA could be reverse transcribed into DNA. The discovery of reverse transcriptase enzymes in the leukoviruses made such views acceptable and if the RNA of an infecting virus is reverse transcribed there seems no reason why the resulting DNA should not potentially be able to "integrate" with the host cell genome.

One of the first benefits arising from this discovery

was the clarification of the problem of the mechanism of the
action of the RNA of tumour viruses as already discussed.
Although this mechanism is in many ways reminiscent of the
slow virus process. the development of cancer cells as the
end product is another variation.   Why some DNA viruses
bring about the replication of viral DNA - sometimes with
the suppression of host DNA synthesis - while others act as
tumor inducers with the ultimate production of modified host
DNA, and some RNA viruses do not replicate as such, but by
going through a DNA phase also stimulate rapid synthesis of
host-like DNA is an interesting if unanswerable question.

It may be useful here to draw an analogy between the
organization of a single cell and that of a complex industrial
corporation.   In such a business structure there is normally
an executive board, comprising several members in whom the
control of all activities are vested and who, after discussion
and agreement, formulate all major policy decisions.   Each
individual member is obviously able to influence the rest,
and some may be more successful in doing so than others.
The decisions are then handed down to management groups in
order that the details necessary for implementation may be
worked out, and specific instructions are then given to
further groups of individuals who actually carry out the
tasks involved.   Although some feed-back is obviously
necessary, this will usually involve requests for such things
as further information and clarification.   Returning to the
cell the executive board is represented by DNA, the management groups by RNA and the final groups by a whole range of
pieces of cellular machinery.   It seems inescapable to conclude that viral DNA (whether arising from reverse transcriptase activity or not) may enter at top level and take its

place on the board.   Its success or failure as an infective
agent presumably depends on the extent to which it can achieve
dominance over its fellow directors.   A new managing director
imposed following the take-over of the company, or a new
powerful individual on the board, could force it to completely
change its direction.   This is analogous to the take-over
of the host cell by a fast-growing virus.   Similarly, a less
powerful member could persuade the board to branch out and
produce a new line of goods while maintaining all the original
products.   In this case the original board retains considerable control over the new member's activities.   This is
analogous to a slow-growing virus.   A modification of the
company's produce would represent a tumour virus while a no
change situation is equivalent to latency.   Since an RNA
can only enter and take part in the activities of the subsidiary groups, the mechanisms for cellular control open to
it must differ fundamentally, and we suggest that only those
of an inhibitory nature can be effective.   Thus 'take-over'
by an RNA virus would primarily involve its ability to prevent or block implementation of the directions handed down
by the board (DNA genome) associated with the much more
limited influence which can be exerted at its own subsidiary
level.   On this view a DNA provirus produced by reverse
transcriptase action which then enters the genome should be
able to constrain its parent RNA to a minor role in the
overall control of the infected cell.

Returning to the virus-host cell complex:  when infection
by an RNA virus is really effective in preventing cellular
DNA from filling its normal regulatory function, it seems
most likely that because the control mechanisms are inhibited
virions will be made at a rate limited only by the capacity

of the existing synthetic machinery and where there is a race
to produce them in sufficient numbers before the decline and
death of the cell.   When an RNA virus is less able to inhibit
normal cell processes it still seems very unlikely that it
will be capable of maintaining infected cells in a sufficiently viable and stable state for the prolonged period necessary
in slow virus replication, yet ultimately destroy its host.
It is much more likely that such an RNA virus will be able
to replicate without causing obvious damage to the host cell.
Such replication without immediate damage is, of course,
characteristic of the persistent viruses.

Where then do we stand on the grouping together of the
slow viruses in relation to the essential criteria of a slow
virus just given, and the definition made earlier which
attempted to differentiate 'slow' from 'persistent' and
'latent' viruses.   It will be recalled that one of the key
requirements called for 'a progressive increase in the
quantity of virus in the infected organ'.   So far as the
four spongiform encephalopathy agents are concerned a progressive increase in infective agent titer in the CNS has
been shown experimentally and this correlates approximately
with the clinical signs.   As has been said, the experimental
evidence on the nature of their core nucleic acid is very
meagre, but DNA seems more probable than RNA.   If this can
be substantiated, then the spongiform agents would meet our
'slow virus' criteria fully.

Of the remaining diseases in Table 1 the causative agent
of PML also appears to fit the various criteria.   It is known
to have a DNA core and, although clinical assessment is often
made very difficult by the other disease processes commonly
associated with it, there is a progressively increasing virus

titer in the CNS and progressive clinical severity.

However visna is clearly an RNA virus and the evidence that SSPE arises in some way from RNA measles virus, is very strong.   To take visna first:   the evidence is that an increased titer of virus is associated with the progression of the disease.   As has been said, however, a reverse transcriptase enzyme system is carried within the virion, and the evidence supports the view that visna RNA replicates by first entering a DNA phase.

Let us then consider the sequence of events which apparently occurs in infections with a leukovirus.   In this group the virion contains the m-RNA strand.   The first product of transcription by the virion reverse transcriptase enzyme system is an RNA-DNA hybrid, from which a ds-DNA is sequentially derived.   At least part of this DNA is covalently linked to host cell DNA.   There is still some controversy over whether both strands of ds-DNA are transcribed to RNA, but it appears most probable that for practical purposes the only strand transcribed in living mammalian cells is the one complementary to m-RNA.   In the case of leukoviruses therefore this DNA- linked pathway produces more virion m-RNA but probably not a v-RNA strand.   Since of course the m-RNA codes directly for the virion proteins, its synthesis leads to the production of more virions;   i.e. to viral replication.   It is not clear why leukoviruses should go through such a relatively complex series of reactions rather than using an RNA-directed RNA polymerase system to shuttle between m- and v-RNA.   Nevertheless this is what seems to occur and it is perhaps important to stress that the principal function of the new DNA is to be a step in the replication process and to become "integrated" into the

host cell genetic material.   From such an integrated form,
the transcription of viral m-RNA and its subsequent translation into proteins is frequently incomplete and viral
replication does not occur.   It therefore appears that the
host cell-provirus complex is able to exert a considerable
degree of control over subsequent events.

Theoretically at least four pathways for such a DNA
provirus appear possible:-

1)   It may be transcribed back into completely functional
     m-RNA giving viral replication.

2)   The end result may be a tumor and this change may or
     may not be associated with viral replication.

3)   It may become latent, probably after chromosomal
     integration, when by definition, replication of the
     virus will cease until and unless reactivation occurs.

4)   If the integration is other than into a chromosome
     structure the provirus DNA may replicate either as the
     core of a new virus, or as a membrane attached viroid
     exhibiting a form of non-structural integration similar
     to that found with the Herpesviruses, or as we have
     postulated for slow viruses in general.

So far as visna is concerned, although some independent
replication of the reverse transcribed DNA cannot be ruled
out, the basic result is multiplication of the original RNA
virus, i.e. pathway 1) above.   Thus the primary function of
the new DNA is to be transcribed into new viral RNA.   It
seems clear therefore that visna will fit our slow virus
criteria if the suggested restraints on replication of a slow
virus DNA are extended to apply to a restricted transcription
of a proviral DNA phase.   However, what appears to be an
essentially similar (if not identical) virus also produces

the tumor-like maedi disease in the lung.    This suggests
that not only is the difference between the pathways RNA
viral core → DNA → RNA virus and RNA viral core → DNA → tumor
a very small one, but also that there must be basic similarities between slow viruses and tumors.

SSPE presents a more difficult problem because even less
is known of the biology of this disease and there is the
obvious problem that the disease resulting from an acute
infection with measles virus is very different from SSPE.
If (like visna) an RNA reverse transcriptase mediated change
takes place, giving a new DNA derived from measles RNA, the
system obviously differs from that of the leukoviruses in
three important ways.    Firstly, like other paramyxoviruses,
the measles virion RNA is the vegetative strand rather than
the messenger.    Secondly the measles virion carries an RNA-
dependent RNA polymerase(s) whose function is to catalyse
the reactions v-RNA → m-RNA → v-RNA.    Thirdly, measles
virions neither carry a reverse transcriptase enzyme system,
nor is there any evidence that measles m-RNA carries the
necessary coding capacity.

As the m-RNA codes for the virion proteins, the combination of the first two processes ends up as measles virus
replication.    During the early stages of measles infection
it seems reasonable to suppose that this is a close coupled
system producing new complete infectious virions.    As the
infection progresses, the immune responses of the host will
begin to eliminate the new virions and also those cells
bearing virion antigens on their surface.    It therefore
seems probable that, as active virus is eliminated, in the
latter stages of the infection some cells will remain which
contain only small transient amounts of viral m-RNA.    Little

is known of the stability of such RNA in isolation and under
normal circumstances it would be expected to disappear,
probably within a few days.   However, we suggest that if, at
this critical period, an adventitious and concurrent infection
with a leukovirus occurs, then the reverse transcriptase enzyme
system from the leukovirus may copy the measles m-RNA to
produce a new proviral DNA.   By analogy with the leukoviruses
it seems probable that only the m-RNA strand will be transcribed and not the measles virion v-RNA.

We must now consider the fate of the measles proviral
DNA in relation to the four possible pathways.   If the new
DNA follows the first alternative pathway and is simply back-
transcribed by host cell enzymes the result would be functional
measles m-RNA.   Although by analogy with both the leukoviruses and cellular m-RNA the complementary DNA strand
would not be transcribed into (measles) v-RNA, the m-RNA
should nevertheless be able to code for the replicase(s)
driving the m-RNA → v-RNA reaction as it does in normal
measles.   However the end result of such a series of
reactions would be measles virions - produced in an abnormally
complex manner, via a DNA intermediate.   These virions
would then be eliminated by the immune response and the
infection would presumably be aborted.   On the other hand,
if there were a faulty initial transcription of the measles
RNA to DNA due, for example, to a lack of specificity of the
reverse transcriptase, then the new m-RNA transcribed from
the proviral DNA would not be an exact copy of the measles
m-RNA, resulting in a failure to complete the original
replication cycle.   In some ways this might appear to be a
probable course of events.   However, by using the correct
techniques, it is possible to recover complete measles virus

from SSPE brain, and this would make a faulty initial reverse
transcription highly improbable.   Consequently there seems
no way in which pathway 1) can explain the sequence of events
taking place in SSPE.

The second pathway (tumor production) does not apply.
Although the third can explain the long delay between the
initial measles infection and the onset of the new disease,
reactivation to give the replication cycle outlined above
takes us no further forward.   The only remaining pathway
then is replication of the proviral DNA, and further, if it
follows the general properties of proviral DNA some form of
integration with the host genome seems inevitable.   If the
integration is other than into the chromosome structure
the proviral DNA may replicate either as the core of a new
virus or as a membrane-attached viroid in the way suggested
above.   This second possibility is more likely since it
seems improbable that proteins originally specified for the
capsid of a measles v-RNA strand would be able to function
in the same way with a proviral DNA.   Association of the
proviral DNA with perhaps a protein derived from a small
segment of the m-RNA, followed by linkage of the complex to
host-cell membranes would bring the system very much into
line with the scrapie agent.   If therefore accurate proviral
DNA was formed initially, but its replication and/or transcription is constrained due to the metabolic integration, the
necessary conditions for the progress of the system as a slow
virus infection have been achieved.

In view of what has been said about control of cellular
events by externally introduced DNA, it seems reasonable that
a proviral DNA replicating in its own right should have little
difficulty in blocking or turning off the sequence of events

which would lead to the re-establishment of measles virions, under the prevailing circumstances at least. There seem two obvious possibilities. Either the new DNA-host cell complex simply turns off the translation of that part of the m-RNA which codes for the polymerase. Or, if the enzyme is produced it is prevented from carrying out its normal function. The experimental observation that complete measles virus can be recovered from SSPE brain by for example co-cultivation with highly permissive cell lines is then readily explained. All that would be needed is a loosening of the control of the proviral DNA over the host cell complex thus permitting the re-establishment of the normal m-RNA → v-RNA measles system. This may well explain the difficulties in transmitting SSPE or similarly based diseases. If the pro-viral DNA or the putative slow virus based on it was unable to establish itself in the new host it would seem very probable that attempts to transmit SSPE will end simply in the development of measles, and as has been indicated this has almost invariably been the result in practice.

Fig. 5

A summary of the above proposals is given below.

1.      Establishment of measles infection in the brain.

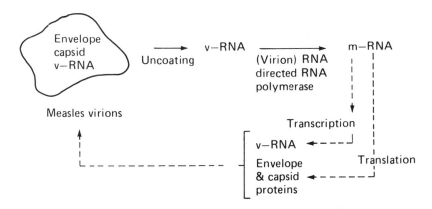

2.      Elimination of measles infection by host defences leaving host brain cells with traces of m—RNA.

3.      Rarely occurring infection at this critical time with a leukovirus carrying a reverse transcriptase enzyme system able to transcribe measles.

$$m-RNA \xrightarrow[\text{transcriptase}]{\text{reverse}} [ss\,DNA] \longrightarrow ds\,DNA$$

4.      Non-structural integration with host cell genome, via attachment to internal host-cell membranes and consequent host restraint on replication. The result is a new slow virus-host cell complex able to turn off the measles m—RNA → v-RNA reaction, thus inhibiting the formation of new measles virions, but allowing the production of measles virion proteins to continue via translation of (measles) m—RNA.

5.      ds—RNA replicates via host polymerase systems thus spreading the new infection and leading to the development of SSPE.

6.      The new system is metastable and under certain circumstances, such as co-cultivation with cells highly permissive for measles virus, the control of the proviral DNA over the host-cell complex may loosen resulting in the re-establishment of the original measles virion system.

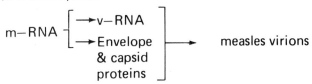

Although there are recent indications that the RNA of
e.g. measles virus may in some circumstances be copied into
a DNA form (82) the suggestion does not previously seem to
have been made that such DNA might become a new infective
agent in its own right.   After our manuscript had been
submitted for publication Zhdanov (81) and Simpson and
Iunuma (74) reported independently that the RNA of such
common viruses as measles and respiratory syncytial virus
could be changed into a DNA form in persistently infected
cell cultures.   Further, and most importantly, that if such
DNA were used to infect (transfect) new cultures the original
RNA virus reappeared.   Zhdanov (81) considered that the
original reverse transcription was brought about by the
presence in the cell cultures of leukoviruses whose virion
reverse transcriptase enzyme systems were able to copy the
RNA of measles and other RNA viruses.   This lends considerable support to the theory on the measles-SSPE relationship
suggested above:   in particular the possibility now seems
very real that DNA prepared from SSPE brain would be capable
of inducing measles virus infection if applied to suitable
cells in culture.

These considerations may also have a bearing on the
relationship of the transmissable Carp agent(s) to multiple
sclerosis and scrapie, which was mentioned in Chapter XI.
Assuming, as before, the basic validity of the published
results, it may be suggested as a possibility that the Carp
scrapie and MS agents are the v-RNA forms of the slow (DNA)
viruses which are the actual etiological agents of the two
diseases.   In this case the Carp agents are to scrapie and
MS what measles is to SSPE.   If the problems of the assay
of the Carp agents could be solved and the whole matter put

on a more sound footing, this suggestion could be tested experimentally. Extraction of DNA from scrapie or MS brain followed by transfection of an appropriate cell system would then be expected to result in the development of the respective Carp agents.

The evidence of the association of similar (Carp) agents with MS and scrapie, itself suggests that the two diseases may be related as Field (40) suggested some years ago. It also supports the views of Adams and Dickinson (7) that many of the disease characteristics of MS could be explained by the underlying presence of a scrapie-like infective agent.

If in fact DNA extracted from MS brain could be shown to transfect cells with the repeatable emergence of any RNA virus this would be prima facie evidence of an underlying viral etiology for MS itself.

As a general summary then, despite the differences already mentioned between the agents causing the spongiform encephalopathies and the other diseases, it does seem practical to bracket them together as a slow virus group, based on the common behaviour of their nucleic acid cores within the infected host and the failure of the host to eliminate them by the use of its normal immune mechanisms.

CHAPTER XIV


THE INCIDENCE OF SLOW VIRUS INFECTIONS


A further common feature of all the slow virus diseases is that they are comparatively rare.  It is possible that there may be occasions when infection occurs, but either fails to develop and is aborted, or does not progress sufficiently to produce clinical symptoms during life. However, as we have said, their very slowness provides a plausible explanation of the apparent failure of the host to protect itself by bringing the viral immune/interferon response mechanisms into play.  This might well favour the alternative suggestion that infection is rare but, when it does occur, a disease state follows, always provided that the host lives long enough.  In the case of PML and SSPE special factors are involved which we have already discussed, while visna-maedi has a high incidence in infected flocks but does not appear to spread readily to surrounding areas.  Once

again however the principal experimental observations bearing
on this question in relation to slow viruses have been derived
from the scrapie agent, although the other spongiform
encephalopathies - kuru in particular - now provide some
clues.

Although the inoculation of normal mice with scrapie
infected mouse tissue is 100% successful in transmitting the
disease, it is almost impossible to demonstrate transmission
by the routes of contagion and infection which would be common
in the human situation.   If normal and scrapie mice are
housed in the same cage for the duration of the disease
process and the normal mice observed for a prolonged period
after the scrapie animals have died, the former rarely
become diseased themselves.   Where disease does develop
the cause is almost always traceable to fighting or to
cannibalism of dead or moribund scrapie animals which had
not been removed from the cages in time.   Transmission from
a scrapie mother to her offspring can occur, but is infrequent.
The most likely reason for this failure of transmission is
the indissoluble association of infectivity with membrane
structures, which means that in all probability tissue fragments from an infected animal would have to be ingested,
particularly in view of the non-infectivity of blood itself.
The recent evidence on the transmission of kuru to primates
also supports the view that even in small doses the disease
can be passed almost 100% successfully by proper inoculation.

The evidence seems, therefore, to favour the conclusion
that these diseases are rare because of the rarity of transmission under normal circumstances - and we have little or
no knowledge of the routes by which such transmission may
occur.   Even the spread of scrapie in sheep is not under-

stood, although suggestions have been made that wild mice
may be the responsible carrier or that placental tissue from
scrapie-infected sheep may be ingested by their fellows.
However the observation that the agent of TME is excreted in
the feces of infected mink, coupled with the fact that mink
are not the natural host species, suggests that in the right
animal and under the right conditions the spongiform
encephalopathy agents may be transmissable by routes common
to other viruses.   Despite this observation, there is little
or no evidence that feces from scrapie mice are infective.
As with so many aspects of the slow viruses, much more work
will be necessary before we can do more than speculate on
the mechanisms of transmission and their relation to the
incidence of slow virus diseases.


SLOW VIRUSES AND THE CENTRAL NERVOUS SYSTEM


     The data in Table 1 suggest that two further parameters
are correlated with slow virus infections.   The first is
the almost complete preponderance of the central nervous
system as the tissue with which disease is associated.
Further, with a single exception, the examples in Table 2
involve the CNS, although of course some of these may eventually be shown not to be slow virus diseases.   Secondly
whereas in the majority of virus infections a rapid replication and disease-producing phase is normally followed by
an equally rapid fall in virus titer and recovery, slow
virus infections produce diseases which almost invariably
end in death.   This is the final result of the 'inexorable
progress' of the build up of the titer of the infective agent.
Thus, to amend slightly the statement of problems made in

the earlier stages of this volume, apart from their slowness
in general why do slow viruses apparently find CNS tissue so
congenial, and when they do attack the CNS why is the outcome
so fatal?   It must be said at the outset that at present
there are no very good answers to these questions and we can
do little more than make a number of comments in the hope
that they are relevant.

To begin with it should be pointed out that the replication of any virus in the tissues of a host animal can only
be detected when some disease process or metabolic change
occurs which can be attributed to it.   The possibility that
there are unrecognised slow virus infections of tissues which
are not associated with any obvious disease has already been
mentioned.   As it is impossible to say how many as yet
unrecognised slow viruses there are, we cannot at present be
certain how far the preponderance of CNS involvement is more
apparent than real.   The obvious possibility is that the
CNS may be more sensitive than other tissues to the disorganisation, which to a greater or lesser extent the presence of
a replicating virus must leave in its wake, and in particular
we must ask whether slow viruses might be particularly
harmful in this situation?

The comment has already been made that although, in
general, adult mammalian tissues synthesise DNA at a low
rate, many remain able to regenerate, and therefore retain a
capability for fast DNA replication.   We must now ask:   has
this any bearing on the rate at which virus replication can
occur within a tissue?   Earlier, in the discussion on normal
DNA synthesis, it was pointed out that the tissues of the
CNS, as well as having an extremely low rate of DNA synthesis
also have a very low regenerative capacity and that in fact

the number of cells per brain decreases during adult life.
In a sense therefore, after reaching maturity - which happens
at a comparatively early stage in the development of the
animal, the brain enters a life-long phase of 'negative DNA
balance'.   This must be almost, if not completely, unique
amongst the major mammalian tissues.   It might be postulated
then that the tissues of the CNS would be more resistant than
most to attempts by invading viruses to 'take them over', or
to any attempt viruses might make to replicate rapidly along-
side the normal metabolic processes.   However, although this
view may be basically correct, as in all attempts to fit slow
viruses into a neat and tidy package, there are aspects of
the problem which obtrude in a rather uncomfortable way.
For example, so far as RNA viruses are concerned, there are a
number which infect the brain and which are associated with
a short incubation period and a relatively rapid rate of
replication.   Possibly the best examples are the so-called
equine encephalitides which are caused by several members of
the alphavirus sub-group of the togaviruses (group A arbo-
viruses).   The infection produced by these viruses in the
CNS follows the normal pattern with a build up of virus
titer in the brain accompanied by a rise in interferon
levels and an immune response, resulting in the elimination
of the virus.   This, incidentally, also makes it clear that
the absence of an immune response and the lack of interferon
production during a slow virus infection of the CNS is not
due to any inherent inability of this tissue to react.   The
alphavirus infection may be sub-clinical or produce enceph-
alitic symptoms followed by death, or recovery with or without
permanent brain damage.   These viruses present no real
problem to the theory because, as has already been stated

normal brain supports a rapid turnover of at least some fractions of cellular RNA.   However there are also DNA viruses -
herpes simplex for example which, so far as can be determined,
infect brain cells (rather than associated connective tissue
for example) and again have short incubation periods and
comparatively rapid replication rates.   A possible explanation is that these viruses have an unusually potent ability
for cell take-over and reorganisation, although it might be
expected that the metabolic inertness of normal brain DNA
would accentuate any tendency viral DNA has to enter the cell
genome.   However, even if this suggestion is on the right
lines, other problems remain in the slow virus-host cell
complex  which are equally difficult to solve.

Does, for example, the regenerative potential of tissue
have any bearing on this relationship?   Let us first consider
scrapie virus and its ability to replicate in the various
tissues, taking liver as an example of one with a high
potential for regeneration.   The experimental results show
that after inoculation with a dose sufficient to infect the
whole animal, the scrapie agent can be detected in the liver,
but seems only to maintain itself at a rather low titer.
In this case at least the scrapie agent seems quite unable
to capitalise on tissue regenerative potential which, as
discussed earlier, is reflected in the ability to return to
a rapid synthesis of host DNA under certain circumstances.
If, in fact slow viruses were able to make use of the regenerative potential of the tissue they infect, there seems no
obvious reason why liver, for example, should not be a
primary focus for the resulting disease rather than brain.
It is of course just possible that slow viruses do have a
rapid replication phase in other tissues which then resolves

by the usual interferon/immune response mechanism, and that
the subsequent slow process in the brain is a secondary
phenomenon.    All that can be said is that while such a
possibility has not been investigated at all thoroughly, the
evidence available would tend not to support it, except in
the probably rather special case of measles-SSPE.    Once
again there is little or no direct evidence one way or
another.    If in fact the slow viruses are transported from
reticuloendothelial tissue, to the brain for example, then
presumably some macrophage or lymphocyte type cells must act
as carriers.    However this is very difficult to reconcile
with the experimentally observed fact that the blood of
scrapie animals is virtually non-infective - even when the
agent titer is high in the reticuloendothelial system itself.

     There are however other aspects of tissue regenerative
ability to be considered.    Let us begin by returning to
the question already asked - 'Is CNS tissue likely to be more
affected than others by the presence of a slow virus?'.
There is a good deal of evidence in tissues such as liver
and muscle than when cells die, or reach a certain stage of
functional disability, they are removed by phagocytosis and
replaced by the normal process of regeneration.    Thus, in
liver, if a slow virus infection were associated with an
insidious process of cell damage, the damaged cells would
tend to be removed as they were formed and any gap left in
the overall functional capacity filled by division of neighbouring cells.    Thus there would be no build up either of
virus or necrotic areas so long as the virus was slow enough.
So far as the fate of virions in cells ingested in this way
is concerned, there are several obvious possibilities.
Depending on their stability, ingested virions might be

wholly or partly degraded with an associated loss in infectivity, whole more resistant agents might well retain their
infectivity and perhaps even replicate within the phagocytic
cells.   In this case they would probably be spread around
the body.   However, so far as the first infected tissue us
concerned, active removal of infected cells would obviously
reduce the titer of the agent, and this would be a further
complication of the previous discussion on the failure of
the scrapie agent to achieve a high titer in liver!

So far as the CNS is concerned, significantly different
factors may well be operating.   Although there is some
disagreement, it seems most likely that the rate of phagocytosis is reduced compared with other tissues because the
entry and exit of phagocytes is impeded by the blood-brain
barrier system.   Also, because of the inability of brain
tissue to regenerate, any infected cells which die and
autolyse, or are phagocytosed, would not be replaced.   The
characteristic 'status spongiosus', seen in spongiform
encephalopathy infections seems to result from the 'disappearance' of neurons, and it might therefore be suggested that
these cells are the primary foci of infection in this group.

It is reasonable then to suppose that such a progressive
loss of tissue, with an associated, progressive, loss of function occurs in the CNS as part of the inexorable process associated with slow virus infection, for two reasons.   Firstly
because of the virtually complete absence of cell regeneration,
particularly of neurons, and secondly because such phagocytosis as occurs in brain seems as likely to cause spread of
infection within the tissue, rather than to eliminate it.

It might perhaps be made clear at this point that the
functional disorganisation and ultimate death of infected

cells envisaged above differs from the more positive 'take over' process discussed earlier.   We believe that most probably the effect of a slow virus infection on CNS cells arises from an insidious, but progressive interference with intracellular mechanisms resulting from the presence of virions or viral components.   Clearly, of course all tissues depend on the integrity of their internal organisation if they are to remain functional.   However, the function of CNS tissue is, to a greater extent than most, critically dependent on the maintenance of a complex pattern of semi-permeable membrane systems, and the immediate availability of large amounts of high energy phosphate compounds.   On general grounds therefore it might be suggested that the intimate binding of scrapie agent to the membrane systems of infected brain cells would be particularly disruptive to their internal organisation.   Further only a comparatively small amount of virus might be required within each cell to cause a significant degree of cellular disfunction. Certainly however the comment has been made that the pathological changes seen in scrapie brain in the terminal stage seem insufficient to account for death.   This also points in the direction of a 'metabolic' death in scrapie and probably other slow virus diseases.

# CHAPTER XV

## CLINICAL ASPECTS OF HUMAN DISEASES CAUSED BY SLOW VIRUSES

One of the problems already discussed is whether one
defines a slow virus disease as a disease caused by a slow
(growing) virus, or as any virus disease with an extended
time interval between initial infection and onset of symptoms.  We believe and have tried to show that the diseases
produced by the slow growing viruses have certain common
properties which differentiate them from the late onset
diseases of persistent virus infections.  This chapter will
therefore summarise the clinical manifestations of the slow
viruses described in the preceeding chapters.  Those diseases
which may have a slow virus etiology will be briefly examined
in the next chapter.  It is not proposed to discuss further
the whole range of diseases caused by latent, persistent and
tumour viruses as this would at least double the size of
this monograph.

CREUTZFELDT-JAKOB DISEASE

The name Creutzfeldt-Jakob (CJ) disease has been used to
describe a group of patients with a somewhat varied range of
neurological and psychiatric symptoms.   In general, the form
of the mental deterioration can be related to the distribution
of the pathological lesion observed at autopsy and Daniel
(see ref. 21) has used this as the basis for a broad classification of the cases into four distinct categories.

1)   Jakob type - This makes up about one third of the reported
     cases and is characterised by severe degeneration of
     neurons in the cortical regions adjacent to the central
     sulcus, in the corpus striatum, thalamus, motor nuclei
     of the brain stem and the spinal cord.   The character-
     istic clinical symptoms are pain and spasticity of the
     limbs, sometimes accompanied by muscular atrophy, with
     mental disturbance which later progresses to a severe
     dementia.   The patient invariably dies between one
     and two years after the onset of symptoms.

2)   Diffuse type - This is the commonest form of CJ
     disease with neuronal degeneration spread diffusely
     throughout the cortex, basal ganglia, thalamus, mid-
     brain, cerebellum and spinal cord.   The clinical
     manifestations mirror the pathological lesions with
     aching of limbs, muscle weakness, ataxia, disorientation
     and dementia developing in all cases.   The duration of
     this form of the disease is in the region of six to nine
     months.

3)   Heidenhain type - In this relatively uncommon form of
     CJ disease the earliest signs are visual disturbances,
     often progressing to early blindness due to destruction

of the neurones in the occipital region.   This is
followed by aching of the limbs, ataxia, disorientation
and dementia with death occurring six to nine months
after onset.

4)    Ataxic form - Severe cerebellar degeneration is the
      characteristic lesion in this rare form of the disease,
      giving ataxia as the most prominent clinical feature.

In addition, there are a number of cases which have
features of more than one of the main categories.   It would
therefore appear that there is a continuous spectrum of
clinical manifestations, in which the four types described
form modal points.   It is not possible to determine from
the analysis of the CJ cases whether the range of symptoms
represents a number of distinct strains of CJ virus or is
due solely to variations in host response.   However, if one
takes into account the uniformity of the clinical picture
in kuru, the existence of several strains of CJ virus
appears to be the most likely explanation.


KURU


Kuru presents a uniform clinical picture quite distinct
from any of the variations of CJ disease, and unknown outside
the Fore ethnic group in New Guinea.   The onset is usually
insidious with the first signs being incoordination of such
skilled movements as the ability to maintain balance on a
single log bridge.   This leads to a progressive locomotor
ataxia, often associated with tremor of the head, trunk and
extremities, which is aggravated by movement or emotional
disturbance and disappears during sleep.   As the disease

advances a confused, agitated state may develop which progresses in the  terminal stage to dementia (if the patient
survives long enough).   In the final stages there is gross
incoordination, muscle weakness and slurring of speech.
There have been no confirmed recoveries from established kuru
although the disease may remain static for long periods with
the patient believing recovery has occurred due to accommo-
dation to the slight physical disabilities present at the
time.   So far as we know, death invariably occurs between
three months and two years after the initial onset.   At post
mortem the body is usually wasted and pneumonia is often the
actual cause of death.   Gross pathological changes in the
brain are rarely found, but there is a typical neuronal
degeneration which is most marked in the cerebellum,
accounting for the severity of the ataxia.


PROGRESSIVE MULTIFOCAL LEUCOENCEPHALOPATHY


    Most cases of progressive multifocal leucoencephalopathy
(PML) are superimposed upon a primary chronic disease which
is often neoplastic and is frequently being treated with
immunosuppressive therapy.   The incidence of PML in
relation to age and sex simply reflects that of the associated
diseases.   In all cases the neurological symptons have an
insidious onset and evolve gradually over a period of several
months.   The most common cerebral symptom is a progressive
hemiparesis which occurs in about 80% of the cases.   Less
common symptoms are dementia, aphasia, hemianopia and hemi-
hypesthesia.   Although all the symptoms indicate a focal
distribution of the brain lesions the characteristic change

shown by electroencephalography is diffuse slow wave activity.
The ultimate death of patients with PML may be due to the
primary disease, the PML or an intercurrent infection.


## SUBACUTE SCLEROSING PANENCEPHALITIS

Subacute sclerosing panencephalitis (SSPE) is a disease
which mainly affects school age children, and which can be
divided into three clinical stages.   There is usually an
insidious onset, first noticed by the children's teachers,
of loss of intellectual powers and psychological disturbances.
The abilities of the patients gradually deteriorate until the
children are no longer able to function adequately in society.
Occasionally, especially in preschool children, the onset may
be abrupt with fever, generalised convulsions and visual
disturbances as the presenting features.   The second stage
is reached in a few weeks or months when the patients become
disorientated, blind and bedfast.   The entire skeletal
musculature is involved in mild myoclonic jerks occurring
from four to twelve times per minute.   The arms and legs are
in flexion contraction and the general condition deteriorates
until the patients are functionally decorticated.   A coma
develops in the third stage, the patients become very
emaciated and usually die of an intercurrent infection.

Remissions lasting from a few weeks to several years
have been recorded in many cases, although in some there is
a relentless downward path from onset to death.   The pattern
of electrical activity in the brain alters from stage to stage
and is of considerable importance in confirming the clinical
diagnosis.

MULTIPLE SCLEROSIS

Multiple sclerosis (MS) is a disease of temperate cli-
mates being most common in Canada, Northern Europe and
Northern USA, where it reaches a prevalence of 60 cases in
every 100,000 population.  The onset is usually acute,
with the symptoms developing over a period of minutes to
hours, or it may be insidious over several months.  In
approximately two thirds of the patients symptoms first
appear between the ages of 20 and 40 years.  It is doubtful
if the disease ever occurs below the age of ten, while an
onset after 60 is virtually unknown.  In most reports the
investigators have found a higher incidence in males than
in females, but in England the reverse is true with the
female to male patient ratio being three to two.  The pre-
dominant symptoms arise from focal lesions of the white
matter and are characterised by weakness of the limbs, incoordination, visual disturbances and parasthesiae.  Other
signs and symptoms more characteristic of lesions in grey
matter such as aphasia, seizures and neurogenic atrophy are
rare.  Mental changes are also a feature of MS and may take
the form of intellectual impairment or, more frequently,
emotional changes.  There is often a reduction in the
efficiency of the control of sphincter activity, while
impotence is also a common symptom.  Following the first
attack the majority of patients show complete remission of
their symptoms, but it is impossible to predict when the
next and subsequent attacks will occur.  The duration of MS
from initial symptoms to death may vary from a few weeks to
over 50 years and the average life expectancy of the fatal
cases has been calculated at about 20 years.  Five years

after onset, 70% of patients with MS are still in their
employment.    Death is usually due to intercurrent infections
of the respiratory or genitourinary tracts.

Following the primary attack, MS can progress in one of
four general ways.    In a small number of patients the symptoms of the primary attack rapidly progress and terminate in
death after three or four months.    However, the great
majority of patients show an initial period of remission
followed by a recurrence of the severe symptoms, called an
exacerbation.    Once again the patient shows a partial,
or near complete, recovery and the disease goes into
remission.    This sequence of exacerbations followed by
remissions may persist for a considerable period with great
variations in the lengths of the remission phases.    After
each exacerbation, it is found that the overall clinical state
of the patient has deteriorated with respect to the situation
immediately prior to that exacerbation, but shows a dramatic
improvement over the most severe period.    Ultimately this
fluctuating, or acute, type of illness is replaced by a
steady deterioration leading to increasing physical disability
and ultimately death.    The third type of MS is usually called
"chronic" and is indistinguishable from the later stages of
the second type.    That is it never shows a remission phase
and there is an essentially continuous deterioration.    In
the fourth form, the disease either appears to remit
completely after the initial one or two exacerbations or
stabilises to a steady state of mild disability for life.
In these cases the accuracy of the diagnosis may often be
brought into question.

CHAPTER XVI

SLOW DISEASES OF POSSIBLE VIRAL ETIOLOGY

This title embraces a very heterogeneous collection of
illnesses of man, some of which appear to be related to
diseases we have just considered, and all of which, with the
exception of hepatitis, are listed in Table 2.   Schilder's
encephalitis and Devic's syndrome are rare demyelinating
diseases and as they appear to resemble some aspects of MS
they need not concern us further.   The evidence for a viral
etiology for the remaining diseases of the CNS is even more
circumstantial than it is for MS.   However, Millar (see
ref. 41) has suggested that different diseases would result
if a "slow" virus were to affect diffent cells.   For example
Parkinson's disease would arise from involvement of the basal
ganglion, motor neuron disease from the anterior horn cells,
or MS if the oligodendroglial cells were affected.

194

MOTOR NEURON DISEASES

As the name implies this disease is characterised by
muscle weakness and atrophy which is the result of degeneration
of motor neurons.   The lesions may be of the pyramidal fibers,
the anterior horn cells or the cranial motor nerve nuclei and
the type of disease which results depends on the relative
incidence of the degeneration.   Three distinct clinical
syndromes are usually recognised, but intermediate types also
occur.   The most frequent variant is amyotrophic lateral
sclerosis (ALS) in which the principal signs are weakness of
the upper and, to a lesser extent, the lower limbs with
atrophy and fasciculation.   In some ways the pattern of
progressive muscular atrophy is very similar to ALS but here
the disease consists solely of a wasting of the limb muscles.
The final form is chronic bulbar palsy in which the muscles
of the face and mouth are affected.   The disease is always
fatal with the first signs usually appearing in late middle
age (between 50 and 70).   Death normally occurs two to ten
years after the onset of symptoms, although a more protracted
course with static phases is also seen.   ALS has a world-
wide distribution and accounts for about one out of every
1,000 adult deaths.

Analysis of the epidemiology suggests that there is an
infective etiology for the motor neurone diseases.   However
all attempts to transmit the disease to laboratory animals
have proved unsuccessful and there is no evidence implicating
any of the known viruses in the way that measles virus has
been implicated in the etiology of MS.   Transmission of ALS
to rhesus monkeys has been claimed by a group of workers in
the USSR, but serial passage was not achieved, nor is it

generally accepted by other workers that the monkeys actually developed ALS.

## PARKINSONIAN DEMENTIA

Parkinsonian dementia (PD) is a syndrome related to ALS and both occur in very high incidence among the Chamorro people on the Island of Guam.   PD and ALS each account for approximately one in ten of the deaths among adult Chamorro. The histopathological picture of PD shows similarities to motor neuron, Creutzfeldt-Jakob and Alzheimer's diseases. So far attempts to transmit PD to laboratory animals have been unsuccessful.

## PARALYSIS AGITANS

Paralysis agitans or Parkinson's disease is a slowly progressing illness which usually appears during the sixth and seventh decades of life.   There are two main types of the disease, both of which have an insidious onset.   In one the first and dominant symptom is a tremor of the limbs while in the other the principal symptom is muscular rigidity with the tremor causing very little trouble to the patient.   Once again there is no direct evidence for a viral etiology although Millar has reported that a proportion of patients with Parkinson's disease have circulating measles-specific IgM.

## ALZHEIMER'S DISEASE

Alzheimer's disease and the related Pick's disease are

often called presenile dementias and this name accurately
describes the clinical picture as it occurs in patients
between 40 and 60 years of age.   There is also a more than
passing resemblance to Creutzfeldt-Jakob disease although as
yet it has not proved possible to transmit the disease to
chimpanzees or any other animal.   The main histopathological
lesions are the presence of senile (amyloid-rich) plaques
in the brain and generalised cortical atrophy.


HEPATITIS

     There are two quite distinct types of hepatitis, both
of which are of proven viral etiology despite the fact that
in neither case has the causative virus been definitely
identified.   Infective hepatitis is a normal acute disease
and does not concern us here, whereas serum hepatitis has
several characters suggestive of a slow virus disease.   The
causative virus of serum hepatitis has not yet been cultured,
but the disease is associated with a specific serum-carried
particle called Australia antigen or hepatitis associated
antigen (HAA).   The disease is usually spread artificially
by infected blood products and is always severe.   However,
there is evidence which indicates that sub-clinical infections
may occur quite frequently and there is also some evidence
that HAA may be associated with chronic hepatitis.   Despite
the absence of any method of detecting the actual infectious
virus, serum hepatitis appears to be more correctly classified
as a persistent, rather than a slow, virus infection.   Those
who are interested in studying this disease further are
directed to the symposium edited by MacCallum (61).

CHRONIC POLYMYOSITIS

As the name implies, chronic polymyositis is a multifocal degenerative disease of muscle and there may in
addition be involvement of the overlying skin.   The duration
varies from three months to several years, often with a fatal
outcome.   Electron microscopy of affected muscle tissue has
shown the presence of intracytoplasmic inclusions composed of
either tubules similar to paramyxovirus nucleocapsids or
picornavirus-like particles.   The frequency of occurrence
of the inclusions corresponds very well with the degree of
activity of the disease while in one case the same type of
viral-like nucleocapsids were demonstrated over a period of
18 months.   Occasionally intranuclear inclusions have also
been found.   So far it has not proved possible to grow any
infectious virus in vitro and no serological relationship
has been established with any known paramyxovirus.   At
present we cannot say whether the virus-like particles have
any etiological significance and if they do whether they
represent a slow or a persistent infection.

In the course of the description of each of the tabulated slow virus diseases, the comment has been made that it is rare or comparatively rare.   However, it is also becoming very clear that there is an increasing number of diseases - particularly of the central nervous system - in which a slow virus etiology has been shown or implicated.   It seems very possible that the recognised slow virus diseases represent perhaps not quite the tip, but a relatively small fraction of the total iceberg.   We have given some - admittedly speculative - views on why the CNS might be particularly affected by slow virus diseases.   It must also be remembered that the CNS contains a large number of areas, or groups of cells, which perform different functions and that the CNS influences or affects in some way or another practically every bodily function.   Thus one might extend the remarks of Millar to suggest that many, at present obscure, progressive diseases may well result from slow virus attack on the appropriate centers in the CNS.   The first candidates are the possible slow virus diseases in Table 2, but the list is by no means exhaustive.

Thus, although each individual slow virus disease may be comparatively rare, taken together they begin to contribute significantly to the overall mortality.   The known and possible diseases at the present time are responsible for something like 1% of all adult deaths.   Further, the diseases in general are of extended duration, chronic and associated with a progressive loss of mental and/or physical function, leading, in many cases to almost total incapacity before the inevitable end.   Consequently they made a far greater social impact than their incidence might suggest in terms of the suffering of both patients and relatives, and

in the drain on medical and hospital facilities.    Unfortunately, however, the plain truth at the moment is that there
is no known way of even influencing their inexorable course.

REFERENCES

1.    Adams, D. H.    The relationship between cellular
      nucleic acids in the developing rat cerebral
      cortex.    Biochem. J. 98:    636-640, 1966.

2.    Adams, D. H.    The nature of the scrapie agent.
      A review of recent progress.    Path. Biol. 18:
      559-577, 1970.

3.    Adams, D. H.    Studies on DNA from normal and
      scrapie-affected mouse brain.    J. Neurochem.
      19:    1869-1882, 1972.

4.    Adams, D. H. and Bell, T. M.    The relationship
      between measles virus infection and subacute
      sclerosing panencephalitis (SSPE).    Medical
      Hypotheses 2:    55-57, 1976.

5.    Adams, D. H. and Bowman, B. M.    Studies on the
      properties of factors elevating the activity
      of mouse plasma lactate dehydrogenase.
      Biochem. J. 90:    477-482, 1964.

6.    Adams, D. H. and Caspary, E. A.    The nature of the
      scrapie virus.    Brit. Med. J. iii:    173, 1967.

7.    Adams, D. H. and Dickinson, J. P.    Aetiology of
      multiple sclerosis.    Lancet 1:    1196-1199, 1974.

8.    Adams, D. H. and Field, E. J.    A plasma lactic
      dehydrogenase-elevating virus associated with
      scrapie-infected mice.    J. Gen. Virol. 1:
      449-454, 1967.

9.    Adams, D. H. and Field, E. J.    The infective pro-
      cess in scrapie.    Lancet ii:    714-716, 1968.

10.   Alper, T., Cramp, W. A., Haig, D. A. and Clarke, M.
      C.    Does the scrapie agent replicate without
      nucleic acid?    Nature 214:    764-766, 1967.

11.   Alper, T., Haig, D. A. and Clarke, M. C.    The
      exceptionally small size of the scrapie agent.
      Biochem. Biophys. Res. Comm. 22:    278-284, 1966.

12.    Andrewes, C. H. and Pereira, H. G.    Viruses of
       vertebrates.    (3rd edition).    Balliere Tindall,
       London, 1972.

13.    Brown, P. and Gajdusek, D. C.    No mouse PMN leuko-
       cyte depression after inoculation with brain
       tissue from multiple sclerosis or spongiform
       encephalopathies.    Nature 247:  217-218, 1974.

14.    Carp, R. I., Licursi, P. C.,  Merz, P. A. and Merz,
       G. S.    Decreased percentage of polymorphonuclear
       neutrophils in mouse peripheral blood after inoc-
       ulation with material from multiple sclerosis
       patients.    J. Exp. Med. 136:  618-629, 1972.

15.    Casjens, S. and King, J.    Virus assembly.    Ann.
       Rev. Biochem. 44:  555-611, 1975.

16.    Cho, H. J. and Greig, A. S.    Isolation of 14nm
       particles from mouse brain infected with scrapie
       agent.    Nature 257:  685-686, 1975.

17.    Cuille, J. and Chelle, P. L.    La maladie dite
       tremblante du mouton est-elle inoculable?
       C. R. Acad. Sci. Paris 203:  1552-1554, 1936.

18.    Cuille, J. and Chelle, P. L.    La tremblante du
       mouton est-elle determinee par un virus filtrable?
       C. R. Acad. Sci. Paris 206:  1687-1688, 1938.

19.    Cuille, J. and Chelle, P. L.    Transmission experi-
       mentale de la tremblante a la chevre.    C. R. Acad.
       Sci. Paris 208:  1058-1060, 1939.

20.    Dales, S.    Penetration of animal viruses into cells.
       Progr. Med. Virol. 7:  1-43, 1965.

21.    Dick, G. (Ed.)    Host-virus reactions with special
       reference to persistent agents.    J. Clin. Path.
       25:  Suppl. (Royal Coll. Path.), 1972.

22.    Dickinson, A. G., Fraser, H., McConnell, I., Outram,
       G. W., Sales, D. I. and Taylor, D. M.    Extra-
       neural competition between different scrapie agents
       leading to loss of infectivity.    Nature 253:  556,
       1975.

23. Dickinson, A. G., Fraser, H., Meikle, V. M. H. and Outram, G. W. Competition between different scrapie agents in mice. Nature (New Biol.) 237: 244-245, 1972.

24. Dickinson, A. G., Fraser, H. and Outram, G. W. Scrapie incubation can exceed natural lifespan. Nature 256: 732-733, 1975.

25. Dickinson, A. G. and Meikle, V. M. H. Host-genotype and agent effects in scrapie incubation: change in allelic interaction with different strains of agent. Molec. Gen. Genet. 112: 73-79, 1971.

26. Dickinson, A. G., Meikle, V. M. H. and Fraser, H. Identification of a gene which controls the incubation period of some strains of scrapie agent in mice. J. Comp. Path. 78: 293-299, 1968.

27. Dickinson, A. G., Taylor, D. M. and Fraser, H. Depression of polymorph counts by various scrapie agents. Nature 248: 510-511, 1974.

28. Diener, T. O. Potato spindle tuber "virus" IV. A replicating low molecular weight RNA. Virol. 45: 411-428, 1971.

29. Diener, T. O. Similarities between the scrapie agent and the agent of the potato spindle tuber disease. Annals Clin. Res. 5: 268-278, 1973.

30. Diener, T. O., Schneider, I. R. and Smith, D. R. Potato spindle viroid XI. A comparison of the ultraviolet light sensitivities of PSTV, tobacco ringspot virus and its satellite. Virology 57: 577-581, 1974.

31. Diener, T. O. and Smith, D. R. Potato spindle tuber viroid VI. Monodisperse distribution after electrophoresis in 20% polyacrylamide gels. Virol. 46: 498-499, 1971.

32. Diener, T. O. and Smith, D. R. Potato spindle viroid IX. Molecular weight determination by gel electrophoresis of formylated RNA. Virol. 53: 359-365, 1973.

204

33.    Dressler, D.   DNA replication:  portrait of a
       field in mid passage.   In:  25th Symposium,
       Society Gen. Microbiol. (eds. D. C. Burke and
       W. C. Russell), pp.51-76, 1975.

34.    Duffy, P., Wolf, J., Collins, G., DeVoe, A. G.,
       Streeten, B. and Cowen, D.   Possible person
       to person transmission of Creutzfeldt-Jakob
       disease.   New Eng. J. Med. 290:  6921-6922,
       1974.

35.    Eckhart, W.   Oncogenic viruses.   Ann. Rev.
       Biochem. 41:  503-516, 1972.

36.    Eiserling, F. A. and Dickson, R. C.   Assembly of
       viruses.   Ann. Rev. Biochem. 41:  467-502, 1972.

37.    Eklund, C. M., Kennedy, R. C. and Hadlow, W. G.
       Pathogenesis of scrapie virus infection in the
       mouse.   J. Infect. Diseases 117:  15-22, 1967.

38.    Fareed, G. C. and Salzman, N. P.   Intermediates in
       SV40 DNA chain growth.   Nature 238:  274-277,
       1972.

39.    Fenner, F., McAuslan, B. R., Mims, C. A., Sambrook,
       J.  and White, D. O.   The biology of animal
       viruses.   (2nd edition).   Academic Press Inc.,
       New York, 1974.

40.    Field, E. J.   Slow virus infections of the nervous
       system.   Int. Rev. Exp. Pathol. 8:  129-239,
       1969.

41.    Field, E. J., Bell, T. M. and Carnegie, P. R. (eds.)
       Multiple Sclerosis - Progress in Research,
       North Holland Publishing Co., Amsterdam, 1972.

42.    Gajdusek, D. C. and Gibbs, C. J.   Experimental
       subacute spongiform virus encephalopathies in
       primates and other laboratory animals.   Science
       182:  67-68, 1973.

43.    Gardner, S. D., Field, A. M., Coleman, D. V. and
       Hulme, B.   New human papovavirus (B.K.) isolated
       from urine after renal transplantation.   Lancet
       i:  1253-1257, 1971.

44.     Gefter, M. L.   DNA replication.   Ann. Rev. Biochem.
        44:  45-78, 1975.

45.     Gibbons, R. A. and Hunter, G. D.   Nature of the
        scrapie agent.   Nature 215:  1041-1043, 1967.

46.     Gibbs, C. J. and Gajdusek, D. C.   Transmission and
        characterization of the agents of spongiform virus
        encephalopathies:  Kuru, Creutzfeldt-Jakob disease,
        scrapie and mink encephalopathy.   In:  Immunolog-
        ical disorders of the nervous system.   (L. P.
        Rowland, editor), 383-410, Williams and Wilkins,
        Baltimore, 1971.

47.     Gibson, P. E. and Bell, T. M.   Persistent infection
        of measles virus in mouse brain cell cultures
        infected in vivo.   Arch. ges. Virusforsch. 37:
        45-53, 1972.

48.     Hanson, R. P., Eckroade, R. J., Marsh, R. F., ZuRhein,
        G. M., Kanitz, C. L. and Gustafson, D. P.   Suscept-
        ibility of mink to sheep scrapie.   Science 172:
        859-861, 1971.

49.     Hotchin, J. (ed.)   Slow virus diseases:  progress
        in medical virology, vol. 18, S. Karger, Basel,
        1974.

50.     Hunter, G. D., Kimberlin, R. H., Collis, S. and
        Millson, G. C.   Viral and non-viral properties
        of the scrapie agent.   Annals Clin. Res. 5:
        262-267, 1973.

51.     Hunter, G. D., Kimberlin, R. H. and Gibbons, R. A.
        Scrapie:  a modified membrane hypothesis.   J.
        Theoret. Biol. 20:  355-357, 1968.

52.     Kasamatsu, H. and Vinograd, J.   Replication of
        circular DNA in eukaryotic cells.   Ann. Rev.
        Biochem. 43: 695-720, 1974.

53.     Kates, J. and Beeson, J.   Ribonucleic acid synthesis
        in vaccinia virus.   I.   The mechanism of synthesis
        and release of RNA in vaccinia cones.   J. Mol.
        Biol. 50:  1-18, 1970.

54.    Katz, M.,  Rorke, L. B., Masland, W. S., Koprowski,
       H. and Tucker, S. H.   Transmission of an
       encephalitogenic agent from brains of patients with
       subacute sclerosing panencephalitis to ferrets.
       New Eng. J. Med. 279:  793-798, 1968.

55.    Kimberlin, R. H., Walker, C. A. and Millson, G. C.
       Interspecies transmission of scrapie-like diseases.
       Lancet 2:  1309-1310, 1975.

56.    Koestner, A., McCulloch, B., Krakowka, G. S., Long,
       J. F. and Olsen, R. G.   In:  Slow virus diseases.
       (Eds. W. Zeman and E. H. Lennette), The Williams
       and Wilkins Co., Baltimore, pp.86-101, 1973.

57.    Koldovsky, U., Koldovsky, P., Henle, G., Henle, W.,
       Ackermann, R. and Haase, G.   Multiple sclerosis -
       associated agent:  transmission to animals and
       some properties of the agent.   Infection and
       Immunity 12:  1355-1366, 1975.

58.    Latarjet, R., Muel, B., Haig, D. A., Clarke, M. C.
       and Alper, T.   Inactivation of the scrapie agent
       by near monochromatic ultraviolet light.   Nature
       227:  1341-1343, 1970.

59.    Lavelle, G. C.   Multiplicity of scrapie virus in
       infected mouse spleen cells in vivo.   Infection
       and Immunity 7:  918-921, 1973.

60.    Licursi, P. C., Merz, P. A., Merz, G. S. and Carp,
       R. I.   Scrapie-induced changes in the percentage
       of polymorphonuclear neutrophils in mouse periph-
       eral blood.   Infection and Immunity 6:  370-376,
       1972.

61.    MacCallum, F. O. (ed.)   Early studies of viral
       hepatitis.   Brit. Med. Bull. 28:  105-108, 1972.

62.    Marmur, J., Brandon, C., Newhart, S., Ehrlich, M.,
       Mandel, M. and Konvica, J.   Unique properties
       of nucleic acid from B.Subtilis phage SP15.
       Nature New Biol. 239:  68-70, 1972.

63.    Marsh, H. J.   Progressive pneumonia in sheep.
       J. Am. Vet. Med. Assoc. 15:  458-473, 1923.

64.    Millson, G. C., Hunter, G. D. and Kimberlin, R. H.
       Physicochemical nature of the scrapie agent.    In:
       Slow virus diseases of animals and man.    Ed.
       Kimberlin, R. H.    Elsevier, Amsterdam, pp.243-266,
       1976.

65.    Narang, H. K.    An electron microscopic study of the
       scrapie mouse and rat:    further observations on
       virus-like particles with ruthenium red and lanth-
       anum nitrate as a possible trace and negative
       stain.    Neurobiology 4:    349-363, 1974.

66.    Okazaki, R., Okazaki, T., Sakube, K., Sugimoto, K.
       and Sugino, A.    Mechanism of DNA chain growth I.
       Possible discontinuity and unusual secondary
       structure of newly synthesised chains.    Proc. Nat.
       Acad. Sci. U.S. 59:    598-605, 1968.

67.    Outram, G. W., Dickinson, A. G. and Fraser, H.
       Reduced susceptibility to scrapie after steroid
       administration.    Nature 249:    855-856, 1974.

68.    Padgett, B. L., Walker, D. L., ZuRhein, G. M.,
       Ekroade, R. J. and Dessel, B. H.    Cultivation of
       papova-like virus from human brain with progressive
       multifocal leukoencephalopathy.    Lancet 1:
       1257-1260, 1971.

69.    Pattison, I. H.    Resistance of the scrapie agent to
       formalin.    J. Comp. Path. 75:    159-164, 1965.

70.    Rustigian, R.    Persistent infection of cells in
       culture by measles virus.    II. Effect of measles
       antibody on persistently infected HeLa sublines
       and recovery of a HeLa clonal line persistently
       infected with incomplete virus.    J. Bact. 92:
       1805-1811, 1966.

71.    Sigurdsson, B.    RIDA, a chronic encephalitis of
       sheep.    Brit. Vet. J. 110:    341-354, 1954.

72.    Sigurdsson, B., Grimsson, H. and Palsson, P. A.
       Maedi, a chronic progressive infection of sheep's
       lungs.    J. Infect. Dis. 90: 233-241, 1952.

73.    Sigurdsson, B., Palsson, P. A. and Grimsson, H.
       Visna, a demyelinating transmissable disease of

208

sheep.  J. Neuropath. Exp. Neurol. 16:  389-403, 1957.

74.    Simpson, R. W. and Iinuma, M.  Recovery of infectious proviral DNA from mammalian cells infected with respiratory syncytial virus.  Proc. Nat. Acad. Sci. U.S. 72:  3230-3234, 1975.

75.    Sogo, J. M., Koller, T. H. and Diener, T. O. Potato spindle viroid X.  Visualisation and size determination by electron microscopy.  Virology 55:  70-80, 1973.

76.    Spiegelman, S.  Extracellular strategies of a replicating RNA genome.  In a Ciba Foundation Symposium "Strategy of the viral genome", eds. G. E. W. Wolstenholme and M. O'Connor.  Churchill Livingstone, Edinburgh, pp.45-73, 1971.

77.    Temin, H. M.  Mechanism of cell transformation by RNA tumor viruses.  Ann. Rev. Microbiol. 25: 609-648, 1971.

78.    Thormar, H.  Slow infections of the central nervous system.  Z. Neurol. 199:  1-23 and 151-166, 1971.

79.    Weiner, L. P., Herndon, R. M., Narayan, O., Johnson, R. T., Shah, K., Rubinstein, L. J., Preziosi, T. J. and Conley, F. K.  Isolation of a virus related to SV40 from patients with progressive multifocal leukoencephalopathy.  New Eng. J. Med. 286:  385-390, 1972.

80.    Zeman, W. and Lennette, E. H. (eds.)  Slow Virus Diseases, The Williams and Wilkins Co., Baltimore, 1973.

81.    Zhdanov, V. M.  Integration of viral genomes. Nature 256:  471-473, 1975.

82.    Zhdanov, V. M. and Parfanovich, M. I.  Integration of measles virus nucleic acid into the cell genome. Arch. ges. Virusforsch. 45:  225-234, 1974.

83.    ZuRhein, G. M.  Association of papova-virions with a human demyelinating disease (progressive multifocal leukoencephalopathy).  Prog. Med. Virol. 11: 185-247, 1969.

Natural Ecosystem          Man-made ecosystem eg.
eg. herbs, shrubs,            parking lot, factory, house.
forests, grassland.

1) Conserve, stores energy.

2) Produce $O_2$ and consumes
   $CO_2$

3) Filters, detoxicates pollutants.

4) Maintain silence.

5) forms Carbohydrates with
   energy from sun. food.

6) Maintains beauty if not severely
   disturbed.

7) Wildlife.

8) Maintains fertility of the soil.

9)